New Developments in Medical Research

Alopecia

Risk Factors, Treatment and Impact on Quality of Life

NEW DEVELOPMENTS IN MEDICAL RESEARCH

Additional books and e-books in this series can be found on Nova's website under the Series tab.

NEW DEVELOPMENTS IN MEDICAL RESEARCH

ALOPECIA

RISK FACTORS, TREATMENT AND IMPACT ON QUALITY OF LIFE

PIETRO GENTILE
EDITOR

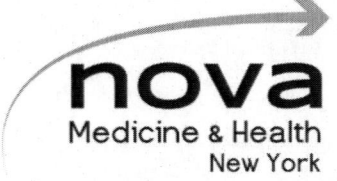

Copyright © 2020 by Nova Science Publishers, Inc.

All rights reserved. No part of this book may be reproduced, stored in a retrieval system or transmitted in any form or by any means: electronic, electrostatic, magnetic, tape, mechanical photocopying, recording or otherwise without the written permission of the Publisher.

We have partnered with Copyright Clearance Center to make it easy for you to obtain permissions to reuse content from this publication. Simply navigate to this publication's page on Nova's website and locate the "Get Permission" button below the title description. This button is linked directly to the title's permission page on copyright.com. Alternatively, you can visit copyright.com and search by title, ISBN, or ISSN.

For further questions about using the service on copyright.com, please contact:
Copyright Clearance Center
Phone: +1-(978) 750-8400   Fax: +1-(978) 750-4470   E-mail: info@copyright.com.

NOTICE TO THE READER

The Publisher has taken reasonable care in the preparation of this book, but makes no expressed or implied warranty of any kind and assumes no responsibility for any errors or omissions. No liability is assumed for incidental or consequential damages in connection with or arising out of information contained in this book. The Publisher shall not be liable for any special, consequential, or exemplary damages resulting, in whole or in part, from the readers' use of, or reliance upon, this material. Any parts of this book based on government reports are so indicated and copyright is claimed for those parts to the extent applicable to compilations of such works.

Independent verification should be sought for any data, advice or recommendations contained in this book. In addition, no responsibility is assumed by the Publisher for any injury and/or damage to persons or property arising from any methods, products, instructions, ideas or otherwise contained in this publication.

This publication is designed to provide accurate and authoritative information with regard to the subject matter covered herein. It is sold with the clear understanding that the Publisher is not engaged in rendering legal or any other professional services. If legal or any other expert assistance is required, the services of a competent person should be sought. FROM A DECLARATION OF PARTICIPANTS JOINTLY ADOPTED BY A COMMITTEE OF THE AMERICAN BAR ASSOCIATION AND A COMMITTEE OF PUBLISHERS.

Additional color graphics may be available in the e-book version of this book.

Library of Congress Cataloging-in-Publication Data

Names: Gentile, Pietro (Plastic surgeon), editor.
Title: Alopecia : risk factors, treatment and impact on quality of life /
  [edited by Gentile Pietro].
Description: New York : Nova Science Publishers, Inc., [2019] | Series:
  Theoretical and applied mathematics | Includes bibliographical
  references and index. |
Identifiers: LCCN 2019058147 (print) | LCCN 2019058148 (ebook) | ISBN
  9781536170085 (paperback) | ISBN 9781536170092 (adobe pdf)
Subjects: LCSH: Alopecia areata.
Classification: LCC RL155.5 .A46 2019 (print) | LCC RL155.5 (ebook) | DDC
  616.5/46--dc23
LC record available at https://lccn.loc.gov/2019058147
LC ebook record available at https://lccn.loc.gov/2019058148

Published by Nova Science Publishers, Inc. † *New York*

CONTENTS

Preface		vii
Chapter 1	Psychological Impact of Alopecia *Nayra Merino de Paz,* *Candelaria Martín-González* *and Mónica Fumero Arteaga*	1
Chapter 2	Androgenetic Alopecia: Diagnosis, Clinical Assessment and Traditional Treatment *Pietro Gentile*	21
Chapter 3	Alopecia Areata: Risk Factors, Treatment and Impact on Quality of Life *Steven K. F. Loo, Kam Lun Hon* *and Alexander K. C. Leung*	29
Chapter 4	A Unique Cocktail of Regenerative Trichology Powered with Right Nutrition - A Novel Approach to Address Hair Disorders *Suruchi Garg and Bhumika Chowdhary*	61
Chapter 5	Growth Factor Rich Therapies for the Treatment of Hair Loss *Megan A. Cole and John P. Cole*	81

Chapter 6	Autologous Micro-Grafts Containing Human Hair Follicle Mesenchymal Stem Cells (HF-MSCs) from Scalp Tissue: Clinical Use in Androgenetic Alopecia *Pietro Gentile*	113
Chapter 7	Platelet Rich Plasma: Clinical Use in Androgenetic Alopecia and Biomolecular Pathway Analysis *Pietro Gentile*	131
Chapter 8	THREE - CO - FAT *Angelo Trivisonno, Giovanni Trivisonno and Filippo Calcagni*	147
Chapter 9	FDA and European Rules Regarding Use of Adipose Derived-Stromal Vascular Cells (AD-SVFs) and Human Follicle Mesenchymal Stem Cells (HF-MSCs) in Hair Re-Growth *Laura Dionisi*	155
Editor's Contact Information		161
Index		163
Related Nova Publications		171

PREFACE

Centuries ago, predicting was an enterprise entrusted to magic and fortune tellers, while today it is the domain of knowledge to which researchers and scientists contribute daily, analyzing and interpreting pathologies, trying to decode the complexity of life, represented by unresolved problems. Regenerating damaged organs and tissues, an act that was also once called magic, is now entrusted to the same scientists and translational surgeons who, through the entrance of the laboratory in the operating room, have allowed us to move from replacement surgery (hair transplant) to regenerative surgery (hair re-growth) with cell therapies and tissue engineering. The passion for Regenerative Plastic Surgery and for the treatment of some pathologies addressed by it, such as Alopecia, has led, over the years, the author and publisher Prof. Pietro Gentile to better investigate, through rigorous scientific studies, the possible new autologous therapies in the treatment of alopecia. This book represents all the latest knowledge in the treatment and prevention of Alopecia, transmitted by all the experts who have decided to contribute to the realization of this work. The visionary idea of this text is therefore to provide the state of the art at the end of the year 2019 in the field of Alopecia.

Chapter 1 - Alopecia is associated to several psychological disorders and impact of quality of life.

Anxiety and depression are the main psychological disorders associated to alopecia. Patients with alopecia areata have shown a high prevalence of anxiety and depression, this suggests that these disorders act as a cause or consequence of it. However, there are few studies performed on other types of alopecias. The authors' case-control studies concluded a higher frequency of anxiety in subjects with alopecia, including subjects with androgenetic alopecia. However, the authors did not find conclusive results regarding depression.

Alexithymia is defined as difficulty being aware of recognizing, differentiating and defining emotions, both of ourselves and others. Several studies have shown a relationship between alexithymia and areata alopecia in recent years. The authors' case-control studies in patients with androgenetic alopecia showed that the patients who consulted for alopecia were found to have higher alexithymia scores than the control subjects, with a statistically significant difference. The patients in the group with alopecia were found to have higher scores for the sub-scales of difficulty to identify the feelings and to verbalize them than the control subjects, with a statistically significant difference. The authors consider that psychological effects of alopecia need a multidisciplinary approach in treatment of these patients.

Chapter 2 - Androgentic Alopecia is the most common, dynamic hair loss disorder, affecting 80% of white men (male-pattern baldness, MPHL) and 40% of women (female-pattern hair loss, FPHL) before age 70. It is important to perform a correct diagnosis of Aandrogenetic Alopecia excluding other causes. Many therapies were suggested to treat this kind of hair loss. The aim of the present chapter is to describe the different analysis useful for AGA diagnosis reporting the effects of traditional therapies, approved by Food and Drug Administration (FDA).

Chapter 3 - Alopecia areata is a systemic autoimmune condition in which hair is lost from the scalp and other areas of the body. People are generally healthy. In some, hair is permanently lost. Risk factors include a family history of the condition. Among identical twins if one is affected the other has about a 50% chance of also being affected. The underlying mechanism involves an immune-mediated destruction of the hair follicle.

Onset is usually in childhood. The condition does not affect a person's life expectancy. In terms of pathophysiology, T cell lymphocytes cluster around affected follicles, causing inflammation and subsequent hair loss. Strong evidence of genetic association with increased risk for alopecia areata was found by studying families with two or more affected members. This study identified at least four regions in the genome that are likely to contain these genes.

The objective assessment of treatment efficacy is very difficult and spontaneous remission is unpredictable. None of the existing therapeutic options are curative or preventive. In cases of severe hair loss, limited success has been achieved by using the corticosteroid injections, or cream. There is no cure for the condition. Efforts may be used to try to facilitate hair regrowth with intralesional corticosteroid injections. Some other medications that have been used are minoxidil, mometasone ointment (steroid cream), irritants (anthralin or topical coal tar), and topical immunotherapy ciclosporin, sometimes in different combinations. Oral corticosteroids may decrease the hair loss, but only for the period during which they are taken, and these medications may cause side effects. A 2008 meta-analysis of oral and topical corticosteroids, topical ciclosporin, photodynamic therapy, and topical minoxidil showed no benefit of hair growth compared with placebo especially with regard to long-term benefits. New biologics and immunomodulating medications have been proposed. Although recent reports demonstrate potential for platelet-rich plasma, ultraviolet radiation, and laser-based modalities in treating alopecia areata, high-quality evidence supporting their efficacy is still lacking. The impact of the disease on quality of life is comparable with other chronic, relapsing skin conditions such as psoriasis and atopic dermatitis, which should be evaluated with validated tools. Effects of alopecia areata are mainly psychological, although these can be severe. Alopecia can be the cause of significant psychological stress. As hair loss can lead to significant changes in appearance, individuals with it may experience social phobia, anxiety, and depression.

Chapter 4 - Hair disorders and their treatments are one of the most intriguing and challenging areas in dermatology practice. Modern dermatology, trichology and regenerative surgery is more result oriented. It aims at restoring the lost hair volume through mesotherapy and platelet rich plasma therapy, or transplanting hormone insensitive -permanent follicular units to introduce new follicles in place of dormant and dead follicles through hair transplant surgery. Considering the huge impact of environmental triggers, like faulty lifestyle and aberrant eating habits, the treatment of hair disorders may not be holistic, unless underlying nutritional deficiencies are corrected. Hair is a neuroendocrine organ; hormone and neuromediator production is in similar lines to that produced by brain, especially in conditions of oxidative and psycho-emotional stress, ultraviolet irradiation, nutritional and sensory stimuli and microbial signals. A sound knowledge in the pathogenesis and diagnosis of hair disorders, correction of underlying nutritional deficiencies and psycho-emotional triggers along with substantial medical treatment is the core approach to the treatment of hair disorders. Regenerative and intervention trichology is a promising, result oriented and ever evolving field in treatment of difficult to treat hair disorders.

Chapter 5 - Traditional approaches to treating hair loss in men and women can be pharmacologic or surgical in nature. Prescription medications like finasteride have associated undesirable side effects including erectile disfunction that may persist long after the treatment is discontinued, and some oral treatments are not recommended for use by female patients. Moreover, topical and oral drug-based treatments require long-term use for continuous effect. In this chapter, the authors will introduce four varieties of alternative treatments that have promising application in the hair regeneration field. Specifically, platelet rich plasma (PRP), amniotic-derived products, adipose-derived products, and exosomes are discussed in terms of their origin, isolation technique, and efficacy in treating hair loss. Of these treatment options, PRP and adipose-derived products have been evaluated most frequently in clinical applications, while amniotic-based products and exosomes have largely been screened at the cellular level in a research capacity. All products have been associated with increased hair growth and induction of the telogen-to-anagen transition.

Chapter 6 - Tissue engineering in hair re-growth aims to develop innovative and not invasive procedures to advance the hair re-growt. The use of autologous micro-grafts containing Human Hair Follicle Mesenchymal Stem Cells (HF-MSCs) has not been adequately considered for hair re-growth in patients affected by Androgenic Alopecia. The aim of the present chapter is to describe the micro-graft preparation with the possibility to isolate the HF-MSCs. In addition the micro-graft infiltration in the scalp using a mechanical and controlled injections as recently published by the author is described. This report would also provide a concise review of recent advances in this field confirming that HF-MSCs contained in micro-grafts may represent a safe and viable treatment alternative against hair loss.

Chapter 7 - Platelet-rich plasma (PRP) has emerged as a new treatment modality in regenerative medicine,and preliminary evidence suggests that it might have a beneficial role in Androgentic Alopecia (AGA). The safety and clinical efficacy of autologous PRP injections for pattern hair loss were investigated in the last 10 years in randomized, placebo-controlled, half-head group study to compare the hair re-growth with PRP versus placebo. No side effects were reported during treatment. The aim of the present chapter is to describe the PRP preparation with the possibility to analyze growth factors and biomolecular pathway. In addition it is described the PRP infiltration in the scalp using a mechanical and controlled injections as recently published by the author. This report would also provide a concise review of recent advances in this field confirming that PRP may represent a safe and viable treatment alternative against hair loss.

Chapter 8 - In the last decades the adipose tissue has acquired an important role in the regenerative field, including hair re-growth. It is important to choose the best tissue for this purpose and the best procedure. The adipose tissue is not uniform. There are differences in relation to the sites of the body, and even to different depth. The choose of the sites and the depth, morever of the types of cannulas and the products of the fat employed, and the correct plane to inject is considered in this chapter.

Chapter 9 - Treatments for hair re-growth based on new biotechnologies as adipose derived-stromal vascular fraction cells (AD-SVFs) and human follicle mesenchymal stem cells (HF-MSCs) must be established performing detailed anamnesis, therapeutic history (i.e., screening for drugs linked to hair loss), clinical examination, blood test, urinalysis, and trichoscopic highlights evaluating specific exclusion and inclusion criteria. In each case, these strategies must be used respecting the FDA and European rules.

In: Alopecia
Editor: Pietro Gentile

ISBN: 978-1-53617-008-5
© 2020 Nova Science Publishers, Inc.

Chapter 1

PSYCHOLOGICAL IMPACT OF ALOPECIA

Nayra Merino de Paz[1], Candelaria Martín-González[2] and Mónica Fumero Arteaga[1]

[1]Dermamedicin Clínicas, Santa Cruz de Tenerife, Spain
[2]Hospital Universitario de Canarias, La Laguna, Tenerife, Spain

ABSTRACT

Alopecia is associated to several psychological disorders and impact of quality of life.

Anxiety and depression are the main psychological disorders associated to alopecia. Patients with alopecia areata have shown a high prevalence of anxiety and depression, this suggests that these disorders act as a cause or consequence of it. However, there are few studies performed on other types of alopecias. Our case-control studies concluded a higher frequency of anxiety in subjects with alopecia, including subjects with androgenetic alopecia. However, we did not find conclusive results regarding depression.

Alexithymia is defined as difficulty being aware of recognizing, differentiating and defining emotions, both of ourselves and others. Several studies have shown a relationship between alexithymia and areata alopecia in recent years. Our case-control studies in patients with androgenetic alopecia showed that the patients who consulted for alopecia were found to have higher alexithymia scores than the control subjects, with a statistically significant difference. The patients in the group with alopecia were found to have higher scores for the sub-scales of difficulty to identify the feelings and to verbalize them than the control subjects, with a statistically significant difference.

We consider that psychological effects of alopecia need a multidisciplinary approach in treatment of these patients.

Keywords: alopecia, anxiety, depression, alexithymia, psychological, HADS, TAS-20

INTRODUCTION

Alopecia represents a common entity in patients of all genders and ages. The most common form is androgenetic alopecia (AGA) but there are other types such as alopecia areata and cicatricial alopecia. Alopecia is often associated with numerous comorbidities like several autoimmune disorders, polycystic ovarian syndrome, cardiac diseases or psychiatric disorders as well as anxiety or depression (Marks et al. 2019).

Anxiety or depression are particularly prevalent in patients with alopecia. Considering specific forms of alopecia, AGA has been associated traditionally to a higher prevalence of anxiety or depression, particularly in young patients with more extensive scalp involvement (Marks et al. 2019). By the age of 30 years, the mean prevalence of AGA is 30 percent, this rate increases to 50% at fifth decade of life (Tanaka et al. 2018) and 65% to 70% for men over 60 years old (Cash 2001). Psychological disorders are different in both sexes in patients with AGA. Women with AGA showed more psychosocial problems (van der Donk et al. 1991; Cash 2001), perhaps because AGA in women is not expected, or because women are usually more interested in their appearance. In a study with 96 women and 60 men with AGA and 56 female control patients, 52% of the women were very affected, relative to 28% of men. Women with AGA had more anxiety and poor self-esteem relative to control group (Cash, Price, and Savin 1993).

However these findings are also common in men. In a European study with 1536 men who responded a structured survey performed by telephone, 47% reported hair loss and 21% of them feelings of depression (Alfonso et al. 2005). Several authors have studied the prevalence of anxiety and depression in androgenetic alopecia, with mixed results, although all agree that these psychiatric disorders are present to a greater or lesser extent in AGA and even some series describe up to 96.4% of symptoms compatible with depressive symptoms ("unhappy feelings") (Goh 2002).

There are a number factors that can predict more negative psychological impact in men with AGA such as younger age men who are in a romantic relationship, men who are strongly worried about their physical appearance, men with personality disorder or poor self-esteem and men who request treatment for AGA (Cash 2001).

Alopecia areata is a common autoimmune disease and the specific mechanisms that conduce to hair loss are not well known, however, genetic factors, environmental factors or autoimmune conditions maybe play an important role. Several studies have linked alopecia areata with symptoms of depression and anxiety, and actually is not clear if AA is a dermatologic disorder with psychiatric manifestations or a psychiatric disease with dermatologic problems (Ghanizadeh and Ayoobzadehshirazi 2014).

Psychiatric disorders in AA have been described time ago. A study published in 1991 showed that 74% of adult patients presented lifetime psychiatric disorder(s), with higher prevalence rates of major depression (39%) and generalized anxiety disorder (39%) (Colon et al. 1991). These findings were in agreement with the results of other groups such as Ruiz-Doblado et al., who showed a higher prevalence of psychiatric comorbidity (66%, especially depression and anxiety) in 32 patients with a previous diagnosis of alopecia. Brain et al., in a study of thirty-nine patients with AA found that 18% of patients with AA experienced symptoms of depression and 51% of patients with AA showed symptoms of anxiety. These authors also observed that an immunological mechanism may be related to the development of depression in this patients (Bain et al. 2019). Other authors compared patients with AA with a control group and found significant difference between the case and control group regarding the prevalence of depression (p = 0.008) and anxiety (p = 0.003) (Aghaei et al. 2014).

In children and adolescents with a diagnosis of AA the prevalence of anxiety and depression is even higher: in a study conducted with 14 patients (mean age: 11,66 ± 6,08 years) it was found that about 78% of the patients with AA had one or more lifetime psychiatric disorder(s), and that the most common was major depressive disorder (50%) (Ghanizadeh 2008).

Patients with primary cicatricial alopecia also showed emotional impact but there are not many studies evaluating this association, probably because is a less common form of alopecia. Chiang et al. in a study conducted with 105 patients with primary cicatricial alopecia found a significant positive correlation with depression (evaluated by Hospital Anxiety and Depression Scale (HADS) (Chiang et al. 2015).

The literal meaning of alexithymia is "no words for feelings" (Provenient of Greek "Alexis": without words and "fear": emotion). It was coined by Sifneos in 1973. This author, defined alexithymia as the difficulty in identifying and expressing verbally the own feelings; and a poor fantasy internal life (Sifneos 1973).

Several elements from other investigations have been added to the initial definition of Sifneos in order to further extend the meaning of this construction. So, the difficulty in locating their own sensations, thinking without symbols and abstractions, and high rigidity in pre-communicative communication, are features that have been added over the years to define this clinical syndrome (García-Esteve, Núnez, and Valdes 1988).

It is important to point out that alexithymia is not a psychiatric diagnostic category. The investigation done so far seems to indicate that this concept is used to refer to a risk factor for a wide variety of medical conditions, since it can increase the susceptibility to develop them (Baiardini et al. 2011).

In the few studies carried out to date about the prevalence rate of alexithymia, there has been an oscillating prevalence between 8% and 10% among university population; Being more common to find it among men

(Blanchard, Arena, and Pallmeyer 1981). In addition, it seems to emphasize the presence of alexithymia among people with a socio-economic and educational low level (Cerezo et al. 1988).

In the literature, it can be observed how there is a number of studies that have related dermatology with psychological and/or psychiatric disorders; acting the latter ones as triggers or as a result of the different dermatological pathologies. Specifically, the interest in studying alexithymia in various dermatological disorders has been growing. That is the case, in which alexithymia is related to psoriasis; where it was found that compared to the control group, the group of patients with psoriasis showed significant alexithymic characteristics (Talamonti et al. 2016). In another study carried out among adolescent patients in a Tunisian dermatology service they showed some results in which there was a positive correlation between vulgar acne and the presence of depression and alexithymia (Feki et al. 2017). Another dermatological disorders that is also related to alexithymia is areata alopecia. It has been shown that patients with areata alopecia have experienced avoidance of close relationships, poor social support and high alexithymic personality features (Picardi et al. 2003).

For all of the foregoing reasons, it is necessary to evaluate the degree of alexithymia between dermatological patients to be able to carry out a multidisciplinary treatment of it. To measure the presence of alexithymia, different tools can be used. Among the most used are the BIQ and TAS 26 or TAS-20, although there are other instruments such as SSPS, MMPI-AS, MMPI APRQ and projective techniques such as TAT or AT-9. The BIQ (Beth Israel Hospital Psychosomatic Questionnaire) has two versions; The first developed by Sifneos in 1973 contains 21 items, that must be completed by the therapist (Sifneos 1973). Its objectivity is doubtful, since according to the previous experience of the interviewer, emotional responses can be obtained. The second version of 1977 (BIQ2) of Sifneos, Apfel and Frankel deals with a self-assessment scale of 17 items that provides extra information to the patient's interview (Sifneos, Apfel-Savitz, and Frankel 1977). TAS-26 (Toronto Alexithymia Scale) developed in 1985 by Taylor, Ryan and Bagby consists of 26 likert response items of

5 points (Taylor, Ryan, and Bagby 1985). From this scale, in 1993, the revised TAS-20 self-assessment scale arises from Parker, Bagby, Taylor, Endler and Schmitz (Parker et al. 1993). The latter consists of 20 items and shares the type of response with the TAS-26. The maximum score of the TAS-20 is 100 with a cut point for 60 alexithymia. In Spain, a transcultural study has been carried out to find psychometric validity to TAS 20 (Páez et al. 1999). This study carried out in Murcia has shown that the TAS-20 is a reliable tool for measuring alexithymia since it showed a similar validity to the one found in 7 different countries (Germany, the United States, Canada, Spain, Mexico, Belgium and England) (Páez et al. 1999). For results like these, the TAS-20 self-assessed scale for alexithymia, is considered the tool with more reliability and validity for clinical research.

DATA AND METHODS

1. Anxiety and Depression

We designed a study to analyze the prevalence of depression and/or anxiety in patients with alopecia.

The study included 40 patients who consulted because of three different types of alopecias (androgenetic alopecia, telogen effluvium or areata alopecia) in our outpatient clinics, and 40 control subjects without clinical history of consultation or treatments for hair loss. All the patients were older than 16 years old. Both groups were matched in age and sex. They were included consecutively, using the Spanish version of the Hospital Anxiety and Depression Scale (HADS) (Caro Gabalda and Ibañez 1992) (Figure 1). The statistical analysis was performed with the SPSS program version 15.0. Cases of anxiety and/or depression were defined by the presence of 11 or more points in each of the two sub-scales. A score less than or equal to 7 is defined as normal, while if between 8 and 10 is considered doubtful and would require the use of others psychometric instruments.

A1	Me siento tenso/a o nervioso/a.	I feel tense or 'wound up'
D1	Sigo disfrutando de las cosas como siempre	I still enjoy the things I used to enjoy
A2	Siento una especie de temor como si algo malo fuera a suceder	I get a sort of frightened feeling as if something awful is about to happen
D2	Soy capaz de reírme y ver el lado gracioso de las cosas	I can laugh and see the funny side of things
A3	Tengo la cabeza llena de preocupaciones	Worrying thoughts go through my mind
D3	Me siento alegre:	I feel cheerful
A4	Soy capaz de permanecer sentado/a tranquilo/a y relajado/a	I can sit at ease and feel relaxed
D4	Me siento lento/a y torpe	I feel as if I am slowed down
A5	Experimento una desagradable sensación de "nervios y hormigueos" en el estómago	I get a sort of frightened feeling like 'butterflies' in the stomach
D5	He perdido el interés por mi aspecto personal	I have lost interest in my appearance
A6	Me siento inquieto/a como si no pudiera parar de moverme	I feel restless as I have to be on the move
D6	Espero las cosas con ilusión	I look forward with enjoyment to things
A7	Experimento de repente sensaciones de gran angustia o temor	I get sudden feelings of panic
D7	Soy capaz de disfrutar con un buen libro o con un buen programa de radio o televisión	I can enjoy a good book or radio or TV program

Figure 1. Spanish and English items of HADS.

2. Alexithymia in Alopecia Patients

We designed a study to quantify the presence of alexithymia using the validated Spanish version of TAS-20 in alopecia outpatients.

The study included 50 patients with alopecia and 50 control subjects from surgery departments (General Surgery, Ophthalmology and Traumatology). All subjects were consecutively recruited and were screened with TAS-20 (Figure 2). Patients were asked to choose only one option. Statistical analysis was performed using SPSS v15.0. We analyzed the presence of alexithymia in each patient. Cases of alexithymia were defined by the presence of 61 points or more and possible alexithymia was consider if the score was between 52 and 60. Three sub-scales (F1 or "difficulty identifying feelings" and "distinguishing between feelings" and "the bodily sensations of emotional arousal," F2 or "difficulty describing feelings to others" and F3 or "externally-oriented thinking") could be analyzed by TAS-20. We compared the results in alopecia group with the surgery control group. Demographic characteristics (age and gender) and clinical features (surgical referral department and type of alopecia) were included in the statistical analysis.

3. Correlation between Alexithymia and Anxiety-Depression in Alopecia Patients

The aim of this study was to quantify the presence of anxiety and depression measured by the HADS and the prevalence of alexithymia using the validated Spanish version of TAS-20 in alopecia outpatients. We were interested in determinate the correlation between mood disorders and alexithymia in these patients.

F1	A menudo estoy confuso con las emociones que estoy sintiendo
F2	Me es difícil encontrar las palabras correctas para mis sentimientos
F1	Tengo sensaciones físicas que incluso ni los doctores entienden
F2	Soy capaz de expresar mis sentiientos fácilmente
F3	Prefiero analizar los problemas mejor que sólo describirlos
F1	Cuando estoy mal no sé si estoy triste, asustado o enfadado
F1	A menudo estoy confundido con las sensaciones de mi cuerpo
F3	Prefiero dejar que las cosas sucedan solas, sin preguntarme por qué suceden de ese modo
F1	Tengo sentimientos que casi no puedo identificar
F3	Estar en contacto con las emociones es muy importante
F2	Me es difícil expresar lo que siento acerca de las personas
F2	La gente me dice que exprese más mis sentimientos
F1	No sé qué pasa dentro de mí
F1	A menudo no sé por qué estoy enfadado
F3	Prefiero hablar con la gente de sus actividades diarias mejor que de sus sentimientos
F3	Prefiero ver espectáculos simples, pero entretenidos, que dramas psicológicos
F2	Me es difícil revelar mis sentimientos más profundos incluso a mis amigos más íntimos
F3	Puedo sentirme cercano a alguien, incluso en momentos de silencio
F3	Encuentro útil examinar mis sentimientos para resolver problemas personales
F3	Buscar significados ocultos a películas o juegos disminuye el placer de disfrutarlos

Figure 2. Spanish version of TAS-20.

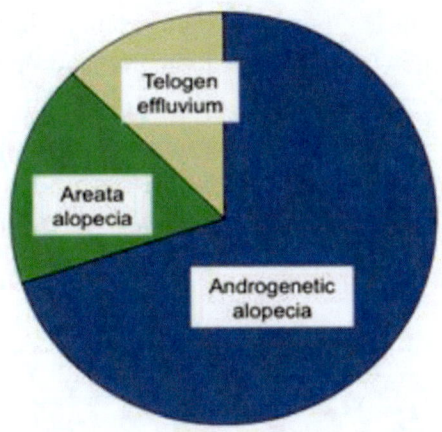

Figure 3. Types of alopecia.

The study included 30 consecutive alopecia patients. All subjects were consecutively recruited and were screened with HADS and TAS-20. Patients were asked to choose only one option in both questionnaires. Statistical analysis was performed using SPSS v15.0.

We analyzed anxiety and depression and/or alexithymia in each patient and the correlation between these entities. Cases of anxiety and depression were defined by the presence of 11 or more points in both sub-scales of HADS. Cases of alexithymia were defined by more than 61 points and possible alexithymia was considered if the score was between 52 and 60 in TAS-20. Patient's demographic characteristics, that were, age, gender and sex, were included in the statistical analysis.

We designed a study to quantify the presence of alexithymia using the validated Spanish version of TAS-20 in alopecia outpatients.

RESULTS

The study to analyze the prevalence of depression and/or anxiety in patients with alopecia showed the following results:

The average age of the patients with alopecia was 40.85 years, being the minimum age 18 and the maximum age 74. The distribution by gender was 82.5% women and 17.5% men in both groups. The most frequent type of alopecia among the patients studied was the androgenetic, followed by alopecia areata and finally telogen effluvium (Figure 3). The item that obtained the highest score in the group Alopecia was 5 ("worrying thoughts go through my mind"), while the 4 ("I can laugh and see the funny side of things") was the one obtained lower score (Figures 4 and 5).

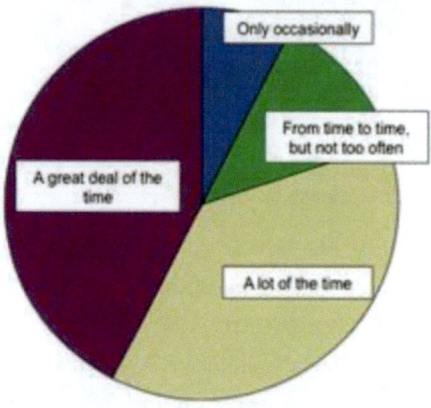

Figure 4. Answers to "worrying thouhts go through my mind" (item 5).

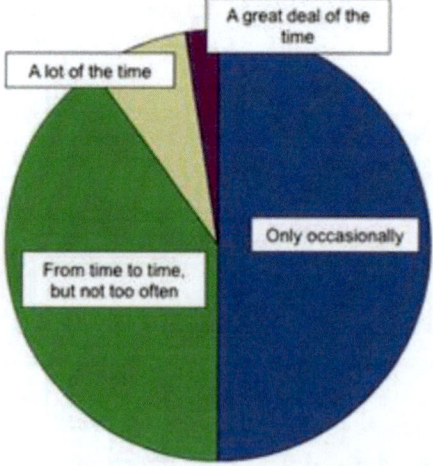

Figure 5. Answers to "I can laugh and see the funny side of things" (item 4).

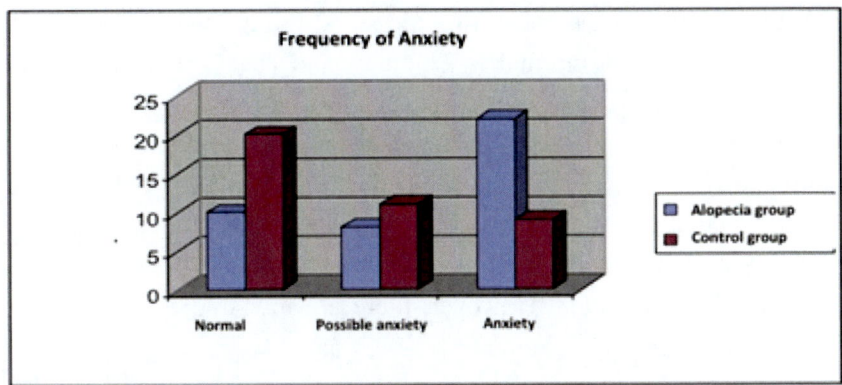

Figure 6. Answers to "I can laugh and see the funny side of things" (item 4).

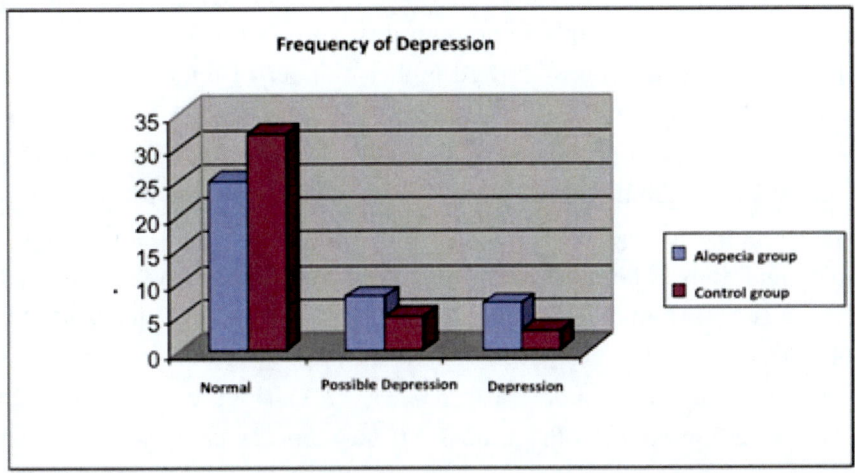

Figure 7. Answers to "I can laugh and see the funny side of things" (item 4).

The mean score for anxiety in the group of patients with alopecia was 11 points, with the maximum score of 21 and the minimum of 4, while the mean score for depression in said group was of 6.22, being the maximum score of 14 and the minimum of 0.

There is a statistically significant difference between the means of overall scores of the anxiety sub-scale among the group of patients with alopecia and the control group (p = 0.005). Also, analyzing the scores in the 3 possible groups (normal, doubtful or case), there is a statistically significant difference between the alopecia group and control group between the subgroups normal (≤7 points) and case (≥11) points) (p = 0.003) (Figure 6).

There are no statistically significant differences between both groups for the scores on the depression sub-scale (Figure 7). Different clinical cases and studies show a high prevalence of anxiety and depression in patients with alopecia areata, suggesting that these disorders can act as cause or consequence of it. However, there are few studies performed on other types of alopecia.

The study to quantify the presence of alexithymia using the validated Spanish version of TAS-20 in alopecia patients showed these results:

Alopecia patient ages were between 18 and 74 years old. Age distribution was comparably in both groups with a similar arithmetic mean (Table 1). Alopecia groups showed higher number of females (80%) than the control group, but the difference was not statistically significant. Alexithymia was more frequent in females (Figure 8). Most of control patients were referred from General Surgery Department (42%) and these patients presented higher scores than those referred from Ophthalmology or Traumatology. The most prevalence type of alopecia was androgenetic alopecia (82%) (Figure 9). Higher number of patients with alexithymia or probable alexithymia have been shown in alopecia group in comparison with control subjects (score ≥61: 6% vs 12%) (Figure 10). Sub-scales scores were similar in both groups. Areata alopecia patients showed the higher prevalence of alexithymia (43%) (Table 2).

The study to determinate the correlation between mood disorders and alexithymia in these patients showed the following results:

Patient's ages were between 18 and 74 years. Sex distribution was 24 females and 6 males. Types of alopecia were androgenetic (83,3%), areata (13,3%) and telogen effluvium (3,3%). There were 13 patients from metropolitan area and 17 live outside, by the countryside. Four patients presented alexithymia and nine were compatible with possible alexithymia (Figure 11). Three of the alexithymia patients were positive for anxiety and depression (75%). Statistical analysis showed a significative correlation between anxiety and alexithymia (p = 0,01) and between depression and alexithymia (p = 0,007). Three alexithymia patients (75%) had androgenetic alopecia. Anxiety and depression were more frequent among patients with androgenetic alopecia.

Table 1. Age distribution in both groups

Age	Maximum	Minimum	Mean	Mode
Control group	69	14	41,52	36
Alopecia group	74	18	39,54	25

Table 2. Alexithymia distribution in relation to the type of alopecia

Type of Alopecia/score	Normal	Probably Alexithymia	Alexithymia
Androgenetic	70,7%	22%	7,3%
Areata	42,9%	14,3%	42,9%
Others	100%	0%	0%

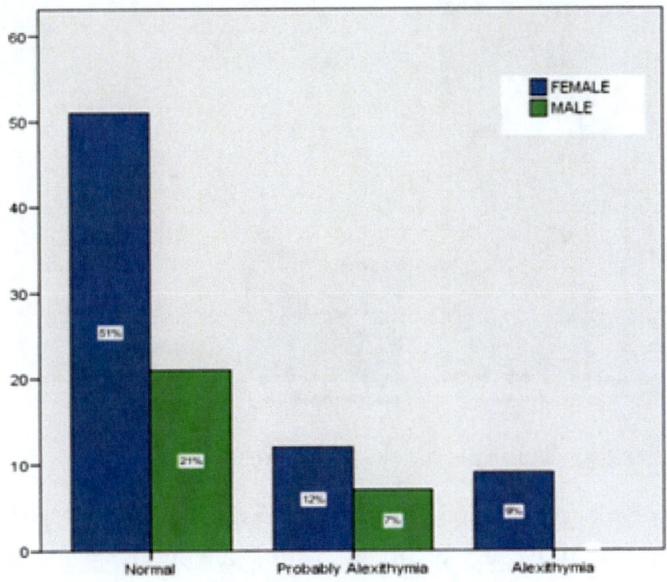

Figure 8. Reation between gender and Alexithymia.

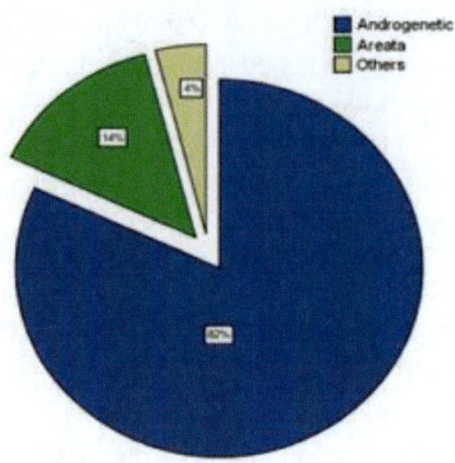

Figure 9. Types of alopecia (Alexithymia case-control study).

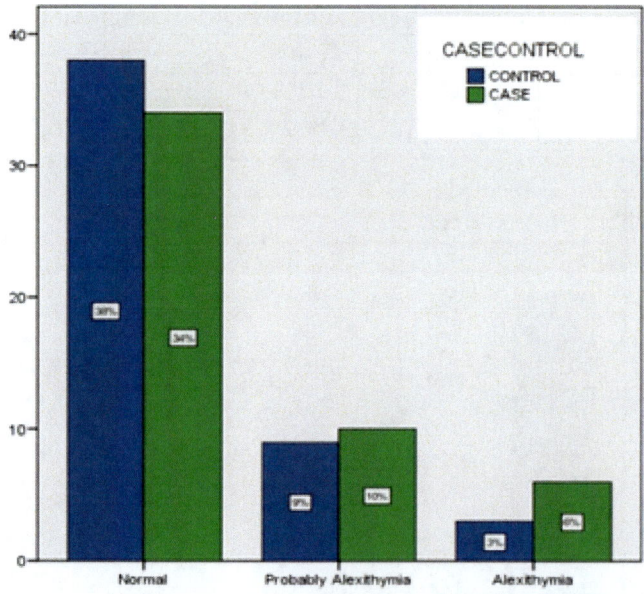

Figure 10. Alexithymia in alopecia cases and control subjects.

The prevalence of anxiety and depression in normal population is around 10-13%. However, in patients with some entities, such as alopecia, this prevalence is higher. In our sample the frequency is 23% for anxiety and 13% for depression (Figures 12 and 13).

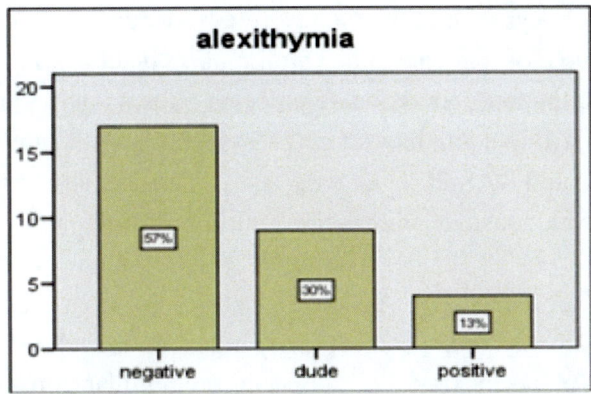

Figure 11. Frequency of Alexithymia.

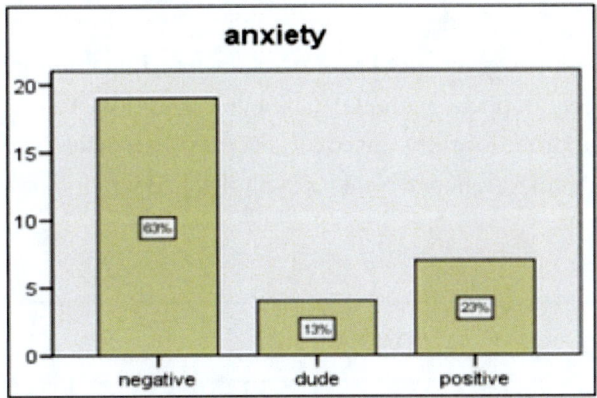

Figure 12. Frequency of anxiety.

There are many studies about alopecia areata and these mood disorders. Therefore, we have found a higher prevalence of alexithymia in patients with alopecia and, to our knowledge this feature has not been described yet.

CONCLUSION

Many dermatological conditions have psychiatric comorbidities. Anxiety and depression have been widely studied (even in our group), but alexithymia is a less well known entity. We have started to study it among different groups of patients. Our preliminary results seem to indicate dermatological patients (in this case alopecia patients) show higher levels. As alexithymia might predispose or be associated with other psychiatric comorbidities, and TAS-20 is an easy test to perform and easy evaluating tool, it might be consider among our multidisciplinary approach to these patients.

With these studies we conclude that there is a possible higher frequency of anxiety in the subjects with alopecia, including subjects with androgenetic alopecia (type of alopecia predominant in our sample). However, we did not find conclusive results in terms of depression, despite of the results of previous studies.

Considering these facts, it would be interesting to include TAS-20 and HADS, quality of life questionaries, or other psychopathology tools in the management of alopecia patients to reach a multidisciplinary approach. This global approach might discover or prevent social or interpersonal relationship dysfunction and other psychological complications in these patients.

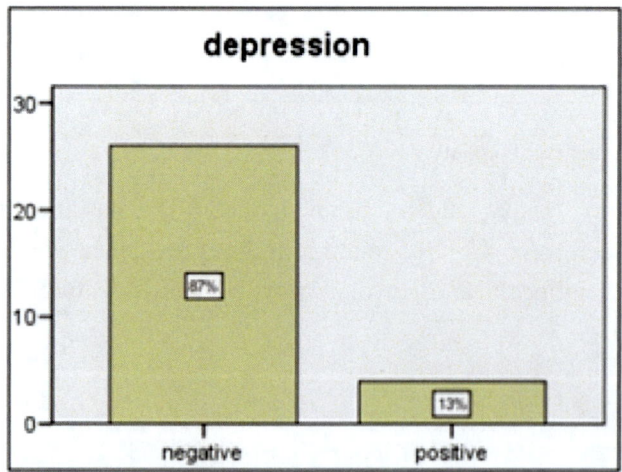

Figure 13. Frequency of depression.

REFERENCES

Aghaei, Shahin, Nasrin Saki, Ehsan Daneshmand, and Bahare Kardeh. 2014. "Prevalence of Psychological Disorders in Patients with Alopecia Areata in Comparison with Normal Subjects." *ISRN Dermatology* 2014: 304370. https://doi.org/10.1155/2014/304370.

Alfonso, Mariola, Hertha Richter-Appelt, Antonella Tosti, Miguel Sanchez Viera, and Marcos Garcia. 2005. "The Psychosocial Impact of Hair Loss among Men: A Multinational European Study." *Current Medical Research and Opinion* 21 (11): 1829-36. https://doi.org/10.1185/030079905X61820.

Baiardini, Ilaria, Silvia Abba, Margherita Ballauri, Giulia Vuillermoz, and Fulvio Braido. 2011. "Alexithymia and Chronic Diseases: The State of the Art." *Giornale Italiano Di Medicina Del Lavoro Ed Ergonomia* 33 (1 Suppl A): A47-52.

Bain, K. A., E. McDonald, F. Moffat, M. Tutino, M. Castelino, A. Barton, J. Cavanagh, et al. 2019. "Alopecia Areata Is Characterised by Dysregulation in Systemic Type 17 and Type 2 Cytokines, Which May Contribute to Disease-Associated Psychological Morbidity." *The British Journal of Dermatology*, April. https://doi.org/10.1111/bjd.18008.

Blanchard, E. B., J. G. Arena, and T. P. Pallmeyer. 1981. "Psychometric Properties of a Scale to Measure Alexithymia." *Psychotherapy and Psychosomatics* 35 (1): 64-71. https://doi.org/10.1159/000287479.

Caro Gabalda, Isabel, and E. Ibañez. 1992. "Escala Hospitalaria de Ansiedad y Depresión. Su Utilidad Práctica En Psicología de La Salud." ["Hospital Anxiety and Depression Scale. Its Practical Usefulness in Health Psychology."] *Boletín de Psicología* 36: 43-69.

Cash, T. F. 2001. "The Psychology of Hair Loss and Its Implications for Patient Care." *Clinics in Dermatology* 19 (2): 161-66.

Cash, T. F., V. H. Price, and R. C. Savin. 1993. "Psychological Effects of Androgenetic Alopecia on Women: Comparisons with Balding Men and with Female Control Subjects." *Journal of the American Academy of Dermatology* 29 (4): 568-75.

Cerezo, P., J. Gándara, L. García, and H Hernández. 1988. "Aspectos Teóricos, Clínicos y Evaluación de La Alexitimia." ["Theoretical and clinical aspects of Alexithymia and its assessment"] *Psiquis: Revista de Psiquiatría, Psicología Médica y Psicosomática* 9 (6-7): 19-29.

Chiang, Y. Z., C. Bundy, C. E. M. Griffiths, R. Paus, and M. J. Harries. 2015. "The Role of Beliefs: Lessons from a Pilot Study on Illness Perception, Psychological Distress and Quality of Life in Patients with Primary Cicatricial Alopecia." *The British Journal of Dermatology* 172 (1): 130-37. https://doi.org/10.1111/bjd.13259.

Colon, E. A., M. K. Popkin, A. L. Callies, N. J. Dessert, and M. K. Hordinsky. 1991. "Lifetime Prevalence of Psychiatric Disorders in Patients with Alopecia Areata." *Comprehensive Psychiatry* 32 (3): 245-51.

Donk, J. van der, J. Passchier, C. Knegt-Junk, M. H. van der Wegen-Keijser, C. Nieboer, E. Stolz, and F. Verhage. 1991. "Psychological Characteristics of Women with Androgenetic Alopecia: A Controlled Study." *The British Journal of Dermatology* 125 (3): 248-52.

Feki, R., R. Sellami, I. Feki, D. Trigui, H. Turki, and J. Masmoudi. 2017. "Association between Depression and Alexithymia in Adolescents with Acne Vulgaris." *European Psychiatry* 41 (April): S437. https://doi.org/10.1016/j.eurpsy.2017.01.432.

García-Esteve, L., P. Núñez, and M. Valdes. 1988. "Alexitimia: Análisis Clínico y Psicométrico de Un Concepto Inicialmente Psicoanalítico." ["Alexithymia: Clinical and Psychometric Analysis of a Firstly Psychoanalytic Concept."] *Psicopatología* 8 (1): 55-60.

Ghanizadeh, Ahmad. 2008. "Comorbidity of Psychiatric Disorders in Children and Adolescents with Alopecia Areata in a Child and Adolescent Psychiatry Clinical Sample." *International Journal of Dermatology* 47 (11): 1118-20. https://doi.org/10.1111/j.1365-4632.2008.03743.x.

Ghanizadeh, Ahmad, and Anaheed Ayoobzadehshirazi. 2014. "A Review of Psychiatric Disorders Comorbidities in Patients with Alopecia Areata." *International Journal of Trichology* 6 (1): 2-4. https://doi.org/10.4103/0974-7753.136746.

Goh, C. L. 2002. "A Retrospective Study on the Characteristics of Androgenetic Alopecia among Asian Races in the National Skin Centre, a Tertiary Dermatological Referral Centre in Singapore." *Annals of the Academy of Medicine, Singapore* 31 (6): 751-55.

Marks, Dustin H., Lauren R. Penzi, Erin Ibler, Athena Manatis-Lornell, Dina Hagigeorges, Mariko Yasuda, Lynn A. Drake, and Maryanne M. Senna. 2019. "The Medical and Psychosocial Associations of Alopecia: Recognizing Hair Loss as More Than a Cosmetic Concern." *American Journal of Clinical Dermatology* 20 (2): 195-200. https://doi.org/10.1007/s40257-018-0405-2.

Páez, Darío, Francisco Martínez-Sánchez, Carmen Velasco, Sonia Mayordomo, Itziar Fernández, and Angélica Blanco. 1999. Validez psicométrica de la escala de alexitimia de Toronto (TAS-20): un estudio transcultural. ["Psychometric validity of the Toronto alexithymia scale (TAS-20): a cross-cultural study."] *Boletín de Psicología*. Vol. 63.

Parker, James D. A., R. Michael Bagby, Graeme J. Taylor, Norman S. Endler, and Paul Schmitz. 1993. "Factorial Validity of the 20-Item Toronto Alexithymia Scale." *European Journal of Personality* 7 (4): 221-32. https://doi.org/10.1002/per.2410070403.

Picardi, A., P. Pasquini, M. S. Cattaruzza, P. Gaetano, G. Baliva, C. F. Melchi, M. Papi, et al. 2003. "Psychosomatic Factors in First-Onset Alopecia Areata." *Psychosomatics* 44 (5): 374-81. https://doi.org/10.1176/appi.psy.44.5.374.

Sifneos, P E. 1973. "The Prevalence of 'alexithymic' Characteristics in Psychosomatic Patients." *Psychotherapy and Psychosomatics* 22 (2): 255-62. https://doi.org/10.1159/000286529.

Sifneos, P. E., R. Apfel-Savitz, and F. H. Frankel. 1977. "The Phenomenon of 'Alexithymia.' Observations in Neurotic and Psychosomatic Patients." *Psychotherapy and Psychosomatics* 28 (1-4): 47-57. https://doi.org/10. 1159/000287043.

Talamonti, Marina, Marco Galluzzo, Stella Servoli, Simone D'Adamio, and Luca Bianchi. 2016. "Alexithymia and Plaque Psoriasis: Preliminary Investigation in a Clinical Sample of 250 Patients."

Dermatology (Basel, Switzerland) 232 (6): 648-54. https://doi.org/10.1159/000453661.

Tanaka, Yohei, Toru Aso, Jumpei Ono, Ryu Hosoi, and Takuto Kaneko. 2018. "Androgenetic Alopecia Treatment in Asian Men." *The Journal of Clinical and Aesthetic Dermatology* 11 (7): 32-35.

Taylor, G. J., D. Ryan, and R. M. Bagby. 1985. "Toward the Development of a New Self-Report Alexithymia Scale." *Psychotherapy and Psychosomatics* 44 (4): 191-99. https://doi.org/10.1159/000287912.

In: Alopecia
Editor: Pietro Gentile

ISBN: 978-1-53617-008-5
© 2020 Nova Science Publishers, Inc.

Chapter 2

ANDROGENETIC ALOPECIA: DIAGNOSIS, CLINICAL ASSESSMENT AND TRADITIONAL TREATMENT

*Pietro Gentile**

Regenerative Surgery, Plastic and Reconstructive Surgery,
University "Tor Vergata", Rome, Italy

ABSTRACT

Androgentic Alopecia is the most common, dynamic hair loss disorder, affecting 80% of white men (male-pattern baldness, MPHL) and 40% of women (female-pattern hair loss, FPHL) before age 70. It is important to perform a correct diagnosis of Aandrogenetic Alopecia excluding other causes. Many therapies were suggested to treat this kind of hair loss.

The aim of the present chapter is to describe the different analysis useful for AGA diagnosis reporting the effects of traditional therapies, approved by Food and Drug Administration (FDA).

---

* Corresponding Author's Email: pietrogentile2004@libero.it.

INTRODUCTION

Androgentic Alopecia is a common, dynamic and chronic hair loss disorder, affecting 80% of white men (male-pattern baldness, MPHL) and 40% of women (female-pattern hair loss, FPHL) before age 70, characterized by progressive hair loss, in which lymphocytes and mast cells have been seen around the miniaturizing follicle detailed in the stem cell-rich lump zone (Alsantali and Shapiro 2009; Price 1999).

Miniaturization of the follicles is characterized by a diminishment of anagen phase, with an improvement in the amount of resting hair follicles, telogen, containing microscopic hairs in a hairless scalp (Gentile 2015, 2017, 2018, 2019). While onset in both males and females may be observed as early as age 18, the progression of hair loss differs markedly between the genders. In men, hair is lost in defined patterns described most commonly by the Norwood and Hamilton scales and often leads to complete baldness; however, FPHL is characterized by diffuse thinning that rarely results in complete baldness.

Several therapies have been proposed for the treatment of AGA, but to date, only oral finasteride, topical minoxidil (2% and 5% solutions or foams), and low level laser have been approved by the US Food and Drug Administration (FDA) to combat MPHL (Gentile 2017).

The aim of the present chapter is to describe the traditional therapy approved by FDA, for AGA treatment, suggesting the protocol to follow to perform the diagnosis of AGA. This chapter would also provide a concise review of recent advances in this field.

METHODS

AGA Diagnosis

AGA Diagnoses must be established performing detailed therapeutic history, clinical examination, blood test and urinalysis, trichoscopic highlights. The grade of AGA in the selected patients must be estimated according to the Norwood- Hamilton (NHs) for male and Ludwig (Ls) scales for females.

In detail, MPHL diagnoses were established on the basis of a detailed medical history (i.e., screening for drugs linked to hair loss), clinical examination, and trichoscopic features (i.e., >20% variability in hair diameter between affected and unaffected areas). Patients were clinically diagnosed with MPHL upon presentation of an increase in miniaturized terminal hair and/or a reduced number of hairs on physical examination and phototrichograms, along with negative hair pull tests. Laboratory ests were performed to exclude alternative causes of hair loss, such as poor nutrition, anemia (i.e., complete blood count, serum iron, serum ferritin, total iron binding capacity, and folic acid), thyroid dysfunction (i.e., triiodothyronine (T3), free T3 (FT3), thyroxine (T4), free T4 (FT4), and thyroid-stimulating hormone (TSH), antithyroid peroxidase, and testosterone), and syphilis (i.e., a venereal disease research laboratory blood test). Urinalysis was used to detect levels of 17-idrocorticosteroid, 17-ketosteroid, dehydroepiandrosterone (DHEA), free cortisol, pregnanetriol (PTL), and testosterone (T) in all participants. Finally, circulating levels of cortisol, dihydrotestosterone (DHT), DHEA, D4-androstenedione, 17-hydroxyprogesterone, 3-α-diol glucuronide, prolactin, and gonadotropins (i.e., FSH and LH) were measured on all patients.

AGA Treatments Approved by FDA

Minoxidil 5% foam is also approved by the FDA for female pattern hair loss FPHL. Finasteride, a selective 5-alpha-reductase inhibitor, has proven largely ineffective in treating FPHL (Price 2000), and, given that the drug may cause abnormalities in the external genitalia of male fetuses, is unsuitable for use by pre-menopausal women. Conversely, daily treatment with 1 mg of finasteride has been shown to reduce serum dihydrotestosterone (DHT) levels by 70% and promote the conversion of hair follicles into the anagen (i.e., growth) phase in male AGA patients

(Drake 1999; Van Neste 2000), though significant improvements in hair density may require up to one year of treatment and users may experience adverse sexual side effects which may persist after the medication is discontinued.

Originally formulated as an antihypertensive, minoxidil is hypothesized to arrest follicular miniaturization and increase anagen duration, both of which counteract the AGA hair loss process (Rousso 2014).

As a result, 60% of users (male or female) show increased hair counts when a 2% topical solution is applied daily (Savin 1987; Whiting, 1992). Higher concentrations may afford greater increases in non-vellus hair densities, but they are not approved for use in FPHL (Levy 2013).

Although the current pharmacotherapies are largely effective in arresting the progression of AGA, they enable only partial hair regrowth at best and require persistent use to maintain the regenerated hair density; hence, many AGA sufferers seek surgical intervention, which is often supplemented with FDA-approved pharmacological therapies in addition to emerging trends in regenerative medicine.

In particular, the contribution of platelets to the inflammatory and healing response has made them an increasingly attractive therapeutic resource in all branches of regenerative medicine owing to the high concentrations of biologically active proteins released from platelet ɑ-granules upon contact with injured tissues.

Recently, the use of low-level laser therapy (LLLT) has been proposed as a treatment for hair loss and to stimulate hair regrowth in AGA. Eleven studies were evaluated by Afifi et al. (Afifi 2017), which investigated a total of 680 patients, consisting of 444 males and 236 females. Nine out of 11 studies assessing hair count/hair density found statistically significant improvements in both males and females following LLLT treatment. Additionally, hair thickness and tensile strength significantly improved in two out of four studies. Patient satisfaction was reported in five studies.

In the other hand, the author published many studies focused on clinical and instrumental evaluation of the PRP effects in patients affected by AGA (Gentile 2015; Gentile 2017; Gentile 2019).

Clinical Assessment of Hair Growth

Assessment of hair growth (HG) may be evaluated in different weeks (Ws) after the treatment, that could be summarized in four phases: T0, before the first treatment, T1 - 3 Ws, T2 - 9 Ws, T3 - 16 Ws, T4 - 23 Ws, T5 - 58 Ws after the last treatment.

The impacts of these therapy on HG must be evaluated using photography (same position, same contrast, same light), the physician's and patient's global evaluation scale, and standardized phototrichograms.

In all partecipants, TA has been marked with a semi-permanent tattoo for the subsequent trichogram.

Phototrichograms can be performed in all TA using Fotofinder videoepiluminescence systems in combination with the Trichoscan digital image analysis.

TrichoScan evaluate hairs per $0.65cm^2$ described as hair count (HC), hairs per cm^2 described as hair density (HD), hair thickness (HT), anagen-to-telogen ratio, and vellus hair-to-terminal hair ratio. All hairs with a thickness > $40\mu m$ are categorized as terminal hairs while those with lesser diameter are categorized as vellus hairs.

AGA Biomolecular Analysis

AGA is characterized by a shorter growth (anagen), which has been associated with increased apoptosis of the hair follicle cells. This result suggests the anagen phase becomes shorter because of differences in the genes regulating apoptosis.

The Wnt pathway has been implicated in the transition from the telogen (resting) to the anagen (growth), and also in the determination of the fate of the stem cells in the hair bulge, which are both dysregulated in balding tissue. Finally, baldness risk loci in the WNT ligand biogenesis and trafficking and Class B/2 (Secretin family receptors) pathways were also associated with height, despite none of the individual loci in these pathways being significant: this suggests a "pathway-wide" effect.

Therefore, baldness shows pathway-specific genetic correlations, which provide a potential biological basis to observed epidemiological correlations. Pathway-specific genetic correlations hold promise in disentangling the shared biological pathways underpinning complex diseases (Pirastu 2017).

RESULTS

Most Recent Clinical Effects of Minoxidil Reported in Literature

In literature, all studies have compared minoxidil 5% with 2%. Although other concentrations (2% to 12.5%) are available. In a recent study of Ghonemy et al. (Ghonemy 2019) they compared 10% versus 5% topical minoxidil in the treatment of AGA. In this double-blinded, placebo-controlled, randomized trial, a total of 90 men with AGA were treated. First group have applied 5% minoxidil solution, second group applied 10% minoxidil solution. Efficacy was evaluated clinically and trichoscopically. After 36 weeks of therapy 5% topical minoxidil (0.47 ± 0.26) (0.59 ± 0.64) was significantly superior to 10% topical minoxidil (0.05 ± 0.13) (0.45 ± 0.74) and placebo (0.01 ± 0.05) (-0.03 ± 0.08) in terms of change from baseline in total vertex and frontal hair mean count respectively.

CONCLUSION

The information reported in this chapter highlights the effects of commercial lotions and traditional therapies in patients affected by AGA but the author feel more the necessity to develop new biotechnology as Platelet rich plasma and autologous cellular therapy as the use of Human Follicle Stem Cells in the AGA treatment improving the quality of life of these patients.

REFERENCES

Afifi, L., Maranda, E. L., Zarei, M., Delcanto, G. M., Falto-Aizpurua, L., Kluijfhout, W. P., Jimenez, J. J. (2017). Low-level laser therapy as a treatment for androgenetic alopecia. *Lasers Surg. Med.,* 49, 27 - 39.

Alsantali, A., Shapiro, J. (2009). Androgens and hair loss. *Curr. Opin. Endocrinol. Diabetes. Obes.,* 16, 246 - 253.

Drake, L., Hordinsky, M., Fiedler, V., Swinehart, J., Unger, W. P., Cotterill, P. C., Thiboutot, D. M., Lowe, N., Jacobson, C., Whiting, D. et al. (1999). The effects of finasteride on scalp skin and serum androgen levels in men with androgenetic alopecia. *J. Am. Acad. Dermatol.,* 41, 550 - 554.

Ghonemy, S., Bessar, H., Alarawi, A. (2019). Efficacy and safety of a new 10% topical minoxidil versus 5% topical minoxidil and placebo in the treatment of male androgenetic alopecia: a trichoscopic evaluation. *J. Dermatolog. Treat.,* 12, 1 - 24.

Gentile, P., Scioli, M. G., Bielli, A., De Angelis, B., De Sio, C., De Fazio, D., Ceccarelli, G., Trivisonno, A., Orlandi, A., Cervelli, V., Garcovich, S. (2019). Platelet-Rich Plasma and Micrografts Enriched with Autologous Human Follicle Mesenchymal Stem Cells Improve Hair Re-Growth in Androgenetic Alopecia. Biomolecular Pathway Analysis and Clinical Evaluation. *Biomedicines,* 8, 7, 2.

Gentile, P., Garcovich, S. (2019). Advances in Regenerative Stem Cell Therapy in Androgenic Alopecia and Hair Loss: Wnt pathway, Growth-Factor, and Mesenchymal Stem Cell Signaling Impact Analysis on Cell Growth and Hair Follicle Development. *Cells,* 16, 8, 5.

Gentile, P., Garcovich, S., Scioli, M. G., Bielli, A., Orlandi, A., Cervelli, V. (2018). Mechanical and Controlled PRP Injections in Patients Affected by Androgenetic Alopecia. *J. Vis. Exp.,* 27, 131.

Gentile, P., Cole, J. P., Cole, M. A., Garcovich, S., Bielli, A., Scioli, M. G., Orlandi, A., Insalaco, C., Cervelli, V. (2017). Evaluation of Not-Activated and Activated PRP in Hair Loss Treatment: Role of Growth

Factor and Cytokine Concentrations Obtained by Different Collection Systems. *Int. J. Mol. Sci.,* 14, 18, 2.

Gentile, P., Garcovich, S., Bielli, A., Scioli, M. G., Orlandi, A., Cervelli, V. (2015). The Effect of Platelet-Rich Plasma in Hair Regrowth: A Randomized Placebo-Controlled Trial. *Stem Cells Transl. Med.,* 4, 11, 1317 - 23.

Levy, L. L., Emer, J. J. (2013). Female pattern alopecia: Current perspectives. *Int. J. Women Health,* 5, 541 - 556.

Pirastu, N., Joshi, P. K., de Vries, P. S., Cornelis, M. C., McKeigue, P. M., Keum, N. Franceschini, N., Colombo, M., Giovannucci, E. L., Spiliopoulou, A. et al. (2017) GWAS for male-pattern baldness identifies 71 susceptibility loci explaining 38% of the risk. *Nat. Commun., 8,* 1584.

Price, V. H. (1999). Treatment of hair loss. *N. Engl. J. Med.,* 341, 964 - 973.

Price, V. H., Roberts, J. L., Hordinsky, M., Olsen, E. A,; Savin, R., Bergfeld, W., Fiedler, V., Lucky, A., Whiting, D. A., Pappas, F. et al. (2000). Lack of efficacy of finasteride in postmenopausal women with androgenetic alopecia. *J. Am. Acad. Dermatol.,* 43, 768 - 776.

Rousso, D. E., Kim, S. W. (2014). A review of medical and surgical treatment options for androgenetic alopecia. *JAMA Facial Plast. Surg.,* 16, 444 - 450.

Savin, R. C. (1987). Use of topical minoxidil in the treatment of male pattern baldness. *J. Am. Acad. Dermatol.,* 16, 696 - 704.

Van Neste, D., Fuh, V., Sanchez-Pedreno, P., Lopez-Bran, E., Wolff, H., Whiting, D., Roberts, J., Kopera, D., Stene, J. J., Calvieri, S. et al. (2000). Finasteride increases anagen hair in men with androgenetic alopecia. *Br. J. Dermatol.,* 143, 804 - 810.

Whiting, D. A., Jacobson, C. (1992). Treatment of female androgenetic alopecia with minoxidil 2%. *Int. J. Dermatol.,* 31, 800 - 804.

In: Alopecia
Editor: Pietro Gentile

ISBN: 978-1-53617-008-5
© 2020 Nova Science Publishers, Inc.

Chapter 3

ALOPECIA AREATA: RISK FACTORS, TREATMENT AND IMPACT ON QUALITY OF LIFE

Steven K. F. Loo[1], MD, Kam Lun Hon[2],*, MBBS, MD and Alexander K. C. Leung[3], MD

[1]The Hong Kong Institute of Integrative Medicine, The Chinese University of Hong Kong
[2]Department of Paediatrics and Adolescent Medicine, The Hong Kong Children's Hospital; Department of Paediatrics & The Hong Kong Institute of Integrative Medicine, The Chinese University of Hong Kong
[3]Department of Pediatrics, The University of Calgary, and the Alberta Children's Hospital, Calgary, Alberta, Canada

ABSTRACT

Alopecia areata is a systemic autoimmune condition in which hair is lost from the scalp and other areas of the body. People are generally

---

* Corresponding Author's Email: ehon@hotmail.com.

healthy. In some, hair is permanently lost. Risk factors include a family history of the condition. Among identical twins if one is affected the other has about a 50% chance of also being affected. The underlying mechanism involves an immune-mediated destruction of the hair follicle. Onset is usually in childhood. The condition does not affect a person's life expectancy. In terms of pathophysiology, T cell lymphocytes cluster around affected follicles, causing inflammation and subsequent hair loss. Strong evidence of genetic association with increased risk for alopecia areata was found by studying families with two or more affected members. This study identified at least four regions in the genome that are likely to contain these genes.

The objective assessment of treatment efficacy is very difficult and spontaneous remission is unpredictable. None of the existing therapeutic options are curative or preventive. In cases of severe hair loss, limited success has been achieved by using the corticosteroid injections, or cream. There is no cure for the condition. Efforts may be used to try to facilitate hair regrowth with intralesional corticosteroid injections. Some other medications that have been used are minoxidil, mometasone ointment (steroid cream), irritants (anthralin or topical coal tar), and topical immunotherapy ciclosporin, sometimes in different combinations. Oral corticosteroids may decrease the hair loss, but only for the period during which they are taken, and these medications may cause side effects. A 2008 meta-analysis of oral and topical corticosteroids, topical ciclosporin, photodynamic therapy, and topical minoxidil showed no benefit of hair growth compared with placebo especially with regard to long-term benefits. New biologics and immunomodulating medications have been proposed. Although recent reports demonstrate potential for platelet-rich plasma, ultraviolet radiation, and laser-based modalities in treating alopecia areata, high-quality evidence supporting their efficacy is still lacking. The impact of the disease on quality of life is comparable with other chronic, relapsing skin conditions such as psoriasis and atopic dermatitis, which should be evaluated with validated tools. Effects of alopecia areata are mainly psychological, although these can be severe. Alopecia can be the cause of significant psychological stress. As hair loss can lead to significant changes in appearance, individuals with it may experience social phobia, anxiety, and depression.

Keywords: alopecia areata, totalis, universalis

INTRODUCTION

Alopecia areata is a chronic immune-mediated inflammatory disease of the hair follicle and typically leads to nonscarring hair loss. (Hon KL, 2008; Hon KL, 2011; Leung, A. K. & Robson, 1993; Mitchell & Krull, 1984; Paus, Nickoloff, & Ito, 2005) It commonly presents with discrete patches of alopecia on the scalp. Other hair-bearing areas may also be affected.

1. Epidemiology

The estimated prevalence of alopecia areata is approximately 0.1 to 0.2%, with a lifetime risk of 2%. (Lee, H. H. et al., 2019) Alopecia areata affects both children and adults but up to 60% are younger than 30 age of age. Both men and women are equally affected. (Villasante, Fricke & Miteva, 2015)

2. Pathophysiology

Hair follicles in normal physiological cycle go through phases of active hair growth (anagen phase), follicular involution (catagen phase), and follicular resting (telogen phase). (Lu et al., 2006) Relative immune privilege of the hair follicle is crucial for this normal physiological process. Several perifollicular autoantigens associated with pigment production are immunogenic. Immune tolerance is established by suppression of the surface molecules required for presenting autoantigens to T lymphocytes and by the generation of local inhibitory signals. (Gilhar, Paus, & Kalish, 2007) In alopecia areata, disruption of the immune privilege triggers the infiltration of mixed inflammatory cells including T cells, mast cells, natural killer cells and dendritic cells towards the pigment producing hair follicle. The perifollicular inflammation leads to the disruption of the normal hair cycle with subsequent hair loss. (Xing et al., 2014)

3. Clinical Manifestations

Alopecia areata most commonly occurs on the scalp but may occur on any hair-bearing area, such as the eyelashes, eyebrows, beard, extremities, or other areas. Patchy alopecia, which manifests as smooth, circular, discrete areas of complete hair loss that develop over a period of a few weeks. The patches may remain discrete or become enlarged and coalesce into various patterns. Hair loss is typically asymptomatic. Occasionally, pruritus or a burning sensation precedes the loss of hair. In a subset of patients, patchy alopecia progresses to alopecia totalis (total loss of scalp hair) or alopecia universalis (loss of all hair over the entire skin surface).

Nail involvement, particularly, nail pitting and trachyonychia, is found in 10 to 30% of children with alopecia areata. (Leung, A. K., Leong, & Barankin, 2019) Nail disease may precede, follow, or coexist with active hair loss. Nail involvement has been associated with greater severity of disease. (Kasumagic-Halilovic & Prohic, 2009)

4. Diagnostic Studies

Dermoscopic examination of the hair and scalp can be helpful for visualizing findings consistent with alopecia areata. (Miteva & Tosti, 2012) Exclamation point hairs, short broken hairs for which the proximal end of the hair is narrower than the distal end, are a common and pathognomonic finding in alopecia areata. Exclamation point hairs are typically found at the edges of expanding patches and can be extracted with minimal traction.

Biopsies are reserved for patients in whom the diagnosis is uncertain despite a careful history and physical examination. Biopsies are taken from the edge of a patch of active hair loss and positioned to include at least a few remaining hairs. The pathologic findings in alopecia areata vary with the acuity of hair loss in the biopsied area. The presence of intense, peribulbar, lymphocytic, inflammatory infiltrates surrounding anagen follicles is characteristic findings in active disease. These infiltrates are often described as resembling swarms of bees. In addition, signs of follicular insult may be seen, such as follicular edema, cellular necrosis, microvesiculation, and pigment incontinence. (Whiting, 2003)

5. Subtypes of Alopecia Areata

Patients with the ophiasis subtype of alopecia areata have band-like alopecia usually at the occipital hairline extending toward the temples. (Hon KL, 2011; Leung, A. K., Adams, & Wong, 2012) The sisaipho subtype occurs in the opposite distribution, causing hair loss in the central part of the scalp and sparing hairs at the margin. "Sudden graying" variant of alopecia areata results in loss of pigmented hairs in short period of time. Acute diffuse and total alopecia, being more common in women, is a variant that presents as diffuse and sudden hair loss. It lasts approximately 3 months and followed by rapid regrowth of the hair. Alopecia areata incognita is characterized by acute diffuse shedding of telogen hairs in the areas and can be confused with telogen effluvium. Biopsy of the scalp is sometimes required for a definitive diagnosis in atypical cases. (Strazzulla et al., 2018) Congenital triangular alopecia, also known as temporal triangular alopecia or Brauer nevus, is a developmental anomaly characterized by an asymptomatic bald patch typically involving the frontotemporal region in a triangular shape. (Leung, Alexander K. C. & Barankin, 2015; Zhao & Zhang, 2018) It is a non-scarring, non-inflammatory and circumscribed form of alopecia. The condition is unilateral in approximately 80% of cases. (Leung, Alexander K. C. & Barankin, 2016; Zhao & Zhang, 2018)

Congenital triangular alopecia is common in Caucasians and rare in blacks. The condition usually manifests at 2 to 5 years of age, with about one-third of cases noticed at birth. (Leung, Alexander K. C. & Barankin, 2015; Zhao & Zhang, 2018) The sex ratio is approximately equal. (Leung, Alexander K. C. & Barankin, 2015; Zhao & Zhang, 2018) Other differential diagnoses include telogen effuvium, androgenic alopecia, cicatricial (scarring) alopecia, post-traumatic alopecia, and secondary syphilis. (Hon KL, 2011)

6. Differential Diagnosis

It is important to differentiate between alopecia areata and trichotillomania. (Hon KL, 2008) In trichotillomania, the morbid impulse to pull out one's own hair, the hairs are broken at various lengths. (Leung, A. K. et al., 2012) In tinea capitis, the diagnosis is suggested by erythema, scaling, and crusting locally on the scalp. Trichorrhexis nodosa is characterized by the development of grayish white nodules on the hair shaft, through which the shaft is easily fractured. (Leung, A. K. et al., 2012) Alopecia is also seen in patients with Netherton syndrome which is characterized by trichorrhexis invaginata ("bamboo hair" or "ball and socket" hair shaft deformity), congenital ichthyosiform erythroderma/ ichthyosis linearis circumflexa, and an atopic diathesis. The hair is typically lusterless, dry, short, sparse, beaded, brittle, and easily broken. When hair breaks at the point of invagination, the appearance simulates a "matchstick" or "golf tee". (Leung A.K., Barankin, & Kin, 2018)

DATA AND METHODS

In this article, we will highlight and discuss the risk factors, current treatment approach and the impact of quality of life in alopecia areata.

RESULTS

1. Risk Factors for Alopecia Areata

1.1. Genetics

There is a strong genetic component in alopecia areata with a 10-fold increased risk in first-degree relatives. In a study of 206 patients with alopecia areata, 20% had a family history of first-degree relative involvement. (Blaumeiser et al., 2006) The importance of genetics is further supported by high concordance rates among identical twins. In a twin study involving 19 sets of monozygotic twins, both twins were affected in 42% of twin sets. (Rodriguez, Fernandes, Dresser, & Duvic, 2010) In contrast, among 31 pairs of dizygotic twins, only 10% shared the disease. Familial cases of alopecia areata, as compared with sporadic cases, are often characterized by a poorer prognosis, more rapid progression, more frequent relapses, and greater resistance to therapy. (Dainichi & Kabashima, 2017) Genome-wide association studies suggested that there were genetic polymorphism in the genes regulating of the innate and adaptive immune systems. (Petukhova et al., 2010) Genomic regions containing the CTLA4, IL-2/IL-21, IL-2RA, and Eos genes, all of which are involved in regulating the regulatory T cells, were identified as susceptibility loci for alopecia areata. (Martinez-Mir et al., 2007) The HLA-DQB1*03 allele is an important marker for susceptibility to alopecia areata. (Megiorni et al., 2011)

1.2. Stress

Stress and psychological disorders are commonly quoted as the etiology of alopecia areata, but the exact pathophysiologic mechanism is still unclear. A recent study reported a high prevalence of pre-existing anxiety and depression among patients with alopecia areata. (Okhovat et al., 2019a) The pathophysiologic mechanism of stress is complex and likely involved at the molecular level with the increase of stress hormones facilitating the immune mediated inflammation. (Yenin, Serarslan, Yönden, & Ulutaş, 2015) Besides, stress could pose an negative impact in the gut microbiota dysbiosis and lead to immune dysregulation. (Moreno-Arrones et al., 2019)

1.3. Comorbidities- Atopy and Autoimmune Disease

Increased risk of alopecia areata in patients with atopy has been reported in various epidemiologic studies. (Huang, Mullangi, Guo, & Qureshi, 2013) The association of alopecia areata with autoimmune diseases such as thyroiditis and vitiligo suggest an autoimmune etiology for this disorder. (Barahmani, Schabath, & Duvic, 2009) Genome-wide association studies (GWAS) revealed shared risk loci between alopecia areata and rheumatoid arthritis, celiac disease, and type I diabetes. (Betz et al., 2015) Systemic autoimmunity may be related to disruption of the immune-privileged status of the hair follicles and lead to the T cell-mediated immune response to the follicular antigens.

2. Management Approach in Alopecia Areata

Treatment of alopecia areata is highly individualized. The management plan is a shared decision with the patients or their parents and involves careful consideration of the patient's goal of treatment and the benefits and risks of treatment. (Messenger, Mckillop, Farrant, Mcdonagh, & Sladden, 2012)

The treatment approach for patients who desire active intervention could be divided according to the extent of involvement: limited patchy scalp hair loss and extensive scalp hair loss.

2.1. Limited Patchy Hair Loss

For patients with small areas of hair loss or hair loss of a recent onset, a "watch-and wait approach is often recommended. (Hon KL, 2011) Intralesional and topical corticosteroids are the preferred initial treatment for patients with persistent patchy alopecia areata. Difficulties in complete coverage of treatment area will be expected if the involvement is too extensive. Children and other patients who cannot tolerate multiple injections can be treated with topical corticosteroids.

2.1.1. Intralesional Corticosteroids

The goal of intralesional steroid injection is to promote regrowth of the hair and to limit hair loss. Injections should be performed on both existing and newly forming patches of alopecia. Although intralesional steroid injection is the most commonly used treatment for alopecia with limited hair loss, there are no randomized trials of intralesional corticosteroids for alopecia areata. One nonrandomized comparative study found regrowth of hair at 33 of 34 sites injected with triamcinolone in 11 patients and at 16 of 25 sites injected with triamcinolone in 17 patients. (Porter & Burton, 1971) Another study reported complete regrowth of hair after four months in 40 out of 62 patients (63%) treated with monthly injections of triamcinolone acetonide. (Kassim et al., 2014) Intralesional triamcinolone acetonide 2.5 to 5 mg/mL is injected into the upper subcutis on the face for eyebrow or beard involvement whereas higher concentrations of 5 to 10 mg/mL could be injected into the upper subcutis on the scalp. Small volumes (<0.1 ml per injection site) are evenly injected into multiple sites with 1 cm apart. The dose per visit is largely determined by the extent of the alopecia and patient tolerance. Generally, the usual total dosage is around 20 mg but less than 40 mg is recommended in one treatment session. (Alkhalifah, Alsantali, Wang, Mcelwee, & Shapiro, 2010b) New growth of hair is usually visible within six to eight weeks. The treatment may be repeated as necessary every four to six weeks and can be discontinued once regrowth is complete. If there is no response after six months, treatment should be discontinued and second line treatments should be considered. (Alkhalifah et al., 2010b)

Local skin atrophy is a major side effect of intralesional steroid injection but usually resolves within a few months. Other cutaneous side effects include telangiectasias and hypopigmentation. The risk for adrenal suppression in patients treated with intralesional corticosteroid injections could be limited by controlling the dose of triamcinolone to less than 40 mg in one treatment session.

2.1.2. Potent Topical Corticosteroids

While potent topical corticosteroids are frequently used to treat alopecia areata, evidence for their effectiveness is limited. Topical corticosteroids could be considered for children and adults who cannot tolerate intralesional injections. In one study, 70 patients with patchy alopecia areata were randomly assigned to topical application of either 0.25% desoximetasone cream or placebo twice daily. After 12 weeks of therapy, there was a trend towards complete regrowth of hair in patients treated with desoximetasone (58 versus 39 percent), although it was not statistically significant. (Charuwichitratana, Wattanakrai, & Tanrattanakorn, 2000) In another study, 105 patients with localized alopecia areata were randomized to a 12-week treatment with betamethasone valerate 0.1% foam applied twice daily, intralesional triamcinolone acetonide (10 mg/mL) administered every three weeks, or topical tacrolimus 0.1% ointment applied twice daily. The authors found >75% hair regrowth in 54, 60, and 0% of patients in these three treatment groups, respectively. (Kuldeep et al., 2011) Preferential use of a potent topical corticosteroid over lower-potency corticosteroids is supported by the findings of a 24-week randomized trial performed on 41 children with alopecia areata involving at least 10% of the scalp surface area. (Lenane et al., 2014) The trial found that twice-daily treatment with clobetasol propionate 0.05% cream for two six-week cycles separated by six weeks was more effective for decreasing the area of scalp hair loss than hydrocortisone 1% cream administered via the same regimen. After 24 weeks, 85% of children treated with clobetasol propionate had at least a 50% reduction in the surface area with hair loss, compared with only 33% of children treated with hydrocortisone.

The response to treatment with topical corticosteroid should be evaluated after three months. Topical corticosteroid should be discontinued if patients do not have hair regrowth. For patients who have hair regrowth, the frequency of application could be tapered off gradually. Similar to intralesional corticosteroids, side effects of topical therapy include local skin atrophy, telangiectasias, hypopigmentation, and adrenal suppression

2.2. Extensive Hair Loss

Topical immunotherapy is the preferred first-line treatment for patients with extensive disease of the scalp. Concomitant intralesional and topical corticosteroid therapy could be used as adjuvant therapy for the strategic sites such as frontal hairline or eyebrows. Systemic glucocorticoids are occasionally used for temporarily slowing rapid, extensive hair loss, but side effects limit their use.

2.2.1. Topical Immunotherapy

Topical immunotherapy is an effective treatment for patients with extensive or recurrent scalp disease. A potent contact allergen is applied weekly to the scalp. The exact pharmacological action remains unknown, but an immunomodulatory effect on the perifollicular inflammatory cell infiltrate could play a role. (Rokhsar, Shupack, Vafai*, & Washenik, 1998; Wasyłyszyn, Kozłowski, & Zabielski, 2007)

A systematic review and meta-analysis of studies evaluating contact immunotherapy with diphenylcyclopropenone (DPCP) or squaric acid dibutyl ester (SADBE) for patchy alopecia areata, alopecia totalis, and/or alopecia universalis found an overall rate of complete (90 to 100%) hair regrowth in 32.3% of patients. (Lee, S., Kim, Lee, & Lee, 2018) Patients with patchy alopecia areata had better response rates than patients with either alopecia totalis or universalis (25 versus 43% for complete regrowth). Relapse after treatment was common. Recurrence rates among patients not receiving and receiving maintenance immunotherapy for alopecia areata were 49 and 38%, respectively. (Lee, S. et al., 2018)

Topical immunotherapy is most commonly performed with diphenylcyclopropenone (DPCP). DPCP is often favored over squaric acid dibutylester (SADBE) because it is less expensive and more stable in solution. SADBE must be refrigerated. DPCP is degraded by light and should be stored in an amber glass bottle or another protective container.

Topical immunotherapy with DPCP begins with the application of a 2% solution to a small area on the scalp for initial contact sensitization. One to two weeks after the sensitization phase, treatment is started with the application of a 0.001% concentration of DPCP to the whole affected areas. Patients should be instructed to wash off DPCP after 24 to 48 hours. While the DPCP remains on the skin, the treated areas should be protected from sun exposure. Treatments are usually repeated once weekly with slowly increasing concentrations of DPCP to a maximum concentration of 2%. The concentration inducing a mild eczematous change is utilized for all subsequent treatments. (Choe, Lee, Lee, Choi, & Lee, 2018)

Signs of hair growth are expected by approximately three months, and the frequency of treatment is reduced once maximal hair growth is attained. Treatment could be discontinued if there is no response after six months, however, delayed improvement of DPCP therapy has been reported. (Wiseman, Shapiro, Macdonald, & Lui, 2001)

Severe dermatitis is a potential side effect of topical immunotherapy. If a vesicular or bullous reaction occurs, the contact allergen should be washed off from the skin and treatment with a topical corticosteroid should be initiated. Other potential side effects include lymphadenopathy, urticaria, vitiligo, and dyschromia. (Choe et al., 2018) Use in pregnant women is not recommended. (Alkhalifah et al., 2010b)

2.3. Refractory Disease

Systemic therapies are occasionally used for severe alopecia areata. A high likelihood of relapse, limited efficacy data, and the potential adverse effects of these drugs limit their use to refractory cases.

2.3.1. Traditional Systemic Agents

2.3.1.1. Systemic Glucocorticoids

Most patients with extensive hair loss are most appropriately treated with topical immunotherapy and local corticosteroids as initial treatment. However, systemic glucocorticoids are occasionally prescribed as a temporary measure to slow hair loss in patients with rapidly progressing, extensive hair loss. These patients may be subsequently transferred to local corticosteroid therapy or topical immunotherapy. (Alabdulkareem, Abahussein, & Okoro, 1998)

Although systemic glucocorticoids appear to stimulate hair growth, the adverse effects associated with these agents limit the duration of therapy, and recurrence of hair loss frequently occurs after the discontinuation of treatment. Dosage of prednisolone at 1 mg/kg per day with tapering is recommended in both adults and children with tapering over four to six weeks. (Kar, Handa, Dogra, & Kumar, 2005) Evidence of hair regrowth is expected after four to six weeks. (Vañó-Galván et al., 2016)

The efficacy of a prednisone taper was investigated in a prospective study of 32 patients with alopecia areata, including 16 patients with alopecia totalis or universalis. After six weeks, 13 patients (40.6%) achieved at least 50% hair regrowth, including 4 patients (12.5%) with 75 to 99% hair loss at baseline and four patients with alopecia universalis. (Olsen, Carson, & Turney, 1992)

2.3.1.2. Cyclosporine

Data from case series and uncontrolled studies suggest cyclosporine given with or without systemic glucocorticoids can induce hair regrowth in alopecia areata. (Kim et al., 2008) In one series, 10 of 25 men with severe alopecia areata had significant hair regrowth during treatment with cyclosporine (2.5 to 6 mg/kg per day for 2 to 12 months). (Yeo et al., 2015) However, cyclosporine therapy is associated with the potential for serious adverse effects that preclude long-term therapy. (Kim et al., 2008)

2.3.1.3. Methotrexate

A systematic review and meta-analysis of primarily retrospective observational studies suggests there may be benefit of oral methotrexate, particularly when used in adults or in conjunction with systemic glucocorticoids. (Phan, Ramachandran, & Sebaratnam, 2019) Patients were generally treated with doses between 7.5 and 25 mg per week. The pooled rate of good or complete response (at least 50% hair regrowth) was 63%. Initial hair regrowth with methotrexate may be evident after approximately three months, and 6 to 12 months of therapy may be necessary for complete regrowth. However, recurrence appears common upon tapering of methotrexate.

2.3.2. Newer Biologics – Systemics and Topicals

2.3.2.1. Janus Kinase Inhibitors

Janus kinase (JAK) inhibitors have been shown to have promising effect for hair growth in alopecia areata in various case reports and open labeled studies. (Liu, Craiglow, Dai, & King, 2017; Park et al., 2017) Oral tofacitinib is the JAK 1/3 inhibitor that has been most studied for the treatment of alopecia areata. (Ibrahim, Bayart, Hogan, Piliang, & Bergfeld,

2017) Beneficial effect of JAK inhibitor on alopecia areata may result from inhibition of T lymphocyte activation through the modulation of proinflammatory JAK pathway. (Gilhar, Keren, & Paus, 2019) Further study is necessary to confirm the efficacy of this treatment. (Craiglow & King, 2014; Xing et al., 2014)

2.3.2.2. Oral JAK Inhibitors

Regrowth of hair has been shown in patients with alopecia areata during treatment with tofacitinib, an oral JAK inhibitor. A retrospective study of 90 adults with severe alopecia areata (at least 40% scalp hair loss, alopecia totalis, or alopecia universalis) who had stable or worsening disease for at least six months and received oral tofacitinib (5 to 10 mg twice daily) for at least four months showed a favorable result. (Liu et al., 2017) Of the 65 patients with a duration of the current disease episode of 10 years or less, 77% had a clinical response (at least 6% improvement in the Severity of Alopecia Tool [SALT] score) and 58% achieved greater than 50% improvement in the SALT score over 4 to 18 months of treatment. Patients with a disease episode longer than 10 years appeared less likely to respond to treatment; the clinical response rate in this population was 32% (8 of 25 patients). No serious adverse effects occurred during treatment.

Data on the use of oral tofacitinib in children are limited. In a series of four children (ages 8 to 10 years) with refractory alopecia totalis or alopecia universalis treated with oral tofacitinib, two had complete regrowth of scalp hair, one had partial regrowth, and one failed to respond. (Craiglow & King, 2019) Responses occurred within three to six months. The three responders received 5 mg twice daily, and the child who failed treatment received 5 mg once daily, which was subsequently increased to 5 mg twice daily after three months. In another series, partial hair regrowth occurred in all of eight adolescents with alopecia universalis treated with oral tofacitinib 5 mg twice daily for 5 to 18 months. Initial signs of regrowth occurred within the first three months. (Castelo-Soccio, 2017) No adverse events occurred in either series.

Further support for a potential role for JAK inhibitors in the treatment of alopecia areata stems from an open-label pilot study, case series, and case reports describing the use of oral ruxolitinib. (Liu & King, 2019) In the open-label study, 9 of 12 patients (75%) with moderate to severe alopecia areata treated with oral 20 mg of ruxolitinib twice daily for three to six months achieved at least 50% hair regrowth by the end of treatment. (Mackay-Wiggan et al., 2016)

The use of JAK inhibitors is associated with increased risk for infection, including herpes zoster and other serious infections. (Valenzuela et al., 2018) The development of malignancy and laboratory abnormalities has also been reported in patients receiving tofacitinib therapy for other diseases. (Wollenhaupt et al., 2014)

2.3.2.3. Topical JAK Inhibitors

Multiple case series suggest topical formulations of ruxolitinib and tofacitinib may be beneficial in the treatment of alopecia. (Craiglow, Tavares, & King, 2016) A 28-week phase 1 trial in which 16 adults with alopecia universalis applied tofacitinib 2% ointment, ruxolitinib 1% ointment, clobetasol dipropionate 0.05% ointment, or vehicle to one of four randomly assigned alopecic areas of the scalp and eyebrows twice daily found hair regrowth in the treated area in 6, 5, 10, and 0 patients, respectively. (Bokhari & Sinclair, 2018) In addition, in a 24-week, open-label study, hair regrowth occurred in 3 of 10 adults with alopecia areata or alopecia totalis treated with tofacitinib 2% ointment. (Liu, Craiglow, & King, 2018) Case series also showed potential benefit of topical JAK inhibitors in children with alopecia. In the larger series, tofacitinib 2% ointment therapy in 11 children with alopecia areata, alopecia totalis, or alopecia universalis refractory to oral and topical corticosteroids was associated with improvement in the SALT score in 8 children, including 3 children who had sufficient hair regrowth to cover the scalp or conceal residual areas of hair loss. (Putterman & Castelo-Soccio, 2018)

2.3.3. Other Therapeutic Options for Alopecia Areata

2.3.3.1. Topical Prostaglandin Analogues

Topical prostaglandin analogues have been studied for eyelash involvement, but their efficacy remains uncertain. (Ross, Bolduc, Lui, & Shapiro, 2005) The majority of studies of topical prostaglandin analogues, including a 16-week randomized trial of 11 patients, have shown no benefit. (Roseborough, Lee, Chwalek, Stamper, & Price, 2009) However, a nonrandomized, prospective study reported benefit with a longer course of therapy. Of 44 patients with eyelash alopecia treated with latanoprost ophthalmic solution for two years, complete or moderate regrowth occurred in 17.5 and 27.5% respectively. None of the 10 patients in the control group attained similar levels of response. (Coronel-Pérez, Rodríguez-Rey, & Camacho-Martínez, 2010)

2.3.3.2. Topical Minoxidil

Randomized trials of topical minoxidil are limited and some trials do show evidence of benefit in patients with limited alopecia areata. Minoxidil does not appear to be effective in patients with alopecia totalis and universalis. (Price, 1987) Topical minoxidil is used twice daily alone or in combination with intralesional or topical corticosteroids. Use of 5% minoxidil solution is shown to be more effective than the 2% solution and continued application is required to maintain growth. If minoxidil is used, minoxidil should be tried for at least three months before evaluating effectiveness. (Fiedler-Weiss, 1987) Topical minoxidil is generally well tolerated but can lead to unwanted growth of facial hair in approximately 3% of women. (Lucky et al., 2004) Pruritus or dermatitis is an occasional adverse events. (Lucky et al., 2004)

2.3.3.3. Platelet-rich Plasma

Platelet-rich plasma, which contains growth factors that are important for cell proliferation and differentiation and has anti-inflammatory properties, may be beneficial in alopecia areata. In one study, 45 patients with chronic, recurring alopecia areata of at least two years' duration were randomly assigned to intralesional injections of autologous platelet-rich plasma, triamcinolone acetonide, or placebo administered once per month for three months. The authors found that platelet-rich plasma injection was most effective for inducing hair regrowth. (Trink et al., 2013) Platelet-rich plasma therapy also was associated with reductions in symptoms of burning or itching in affected areas. Additional studies are necessary to further validate the findings.

2.3.3.4. Light Based Therapy

Psoralen plus ultraviolet A (PUVA) photochemotherapy involves topical or oral administration of a psoralen, a photosensitizing agent, followed by exposure to ultraviolet A (UVA) light. Several uncontrolled series suggest efficacy rates of 60 to 65%, though with a high relapse rate. (Taylor & Hawk, 1995) Other series have found efficacy rates no higher than might be expected without therapy. (Healy & Rogers, 1993) PUVA photochemotherapy has the potential for long-term adverse effects, including cutaneous malignancy.

Excimer laser emits monochromatic ultraviolet B (UVB) light at a wavelength of 308 nm. Its mechanism of action in alopecia areata is thought to involve the induction of T cell apoptosis. In a few small studies and case reports, treatment with the excimer laser was associated with improvement in patchy alopecia areata of the scalp. (Zakaria, Passeron, Ostovari, Lacour, & Ortonne, 2004) Patients with lesions on the extremities, alopecia totalis, or alopecia universalis have not responded to therapy. (Byun, Moon, Bang, Shin, & Choi, 2015)

2.3.3.5. Cosmetic Options

Some patients who elect to forgo treatment or who have inadequate response to medical therapy could use cosmetic camouflage for persistent scalp, eyebrow, or eyelash hair loss. Wigs, hairpieces, shaving of the scalp, and protein powders, sprays, or lotions designed to make hair appear more full may be helpful for scalp hair loss. Eyebrow tattooing can be helpful for loss of eyebrows. Patients with alopecia of the eyelashes may choose to apply false eyelashes. Education from specialty nurse who is experienced with cosmetic camouflage options will be desirable. (Alsantali, 2011)

3. Quality of Life in Alopecia Areata

The World Health Organization defines quality of life (QoL) as "an individual's perception of their position in life in the context of the culture and value systems in which they live and in relation to their goals, expectations, standards, and concerns." Various instruments have been used in addressing the QoL in patients with alopecia areata. They could be divided into general health related QoL and alopecia areata specific QoL. (Liu, King, & Craiglow, 2016; Okhovat, Grogan, Duan, & Goh, 2017; Rencz et al., 2016)

3.1. General Health Related QoL Instruments

3.1.1. Dermatology Life Quality Index
Self-reported questionnaire composed of 10 questions, assessing effect of skin condition on various aspects of life. Scores range from 0 (no effect on patient's life, high HRQoL) to 30 (extremely large effect on patient's life, poor HRQoL). (Finlay & Khan, 1994)

3.1.2. Skindex
Self-reported questionnaire composed of various number of questions, assessing the degree to which an individual is bothered because of various aspects of skin condition. Scores range from 0 (never bothered, high HRQoL) to 100 (always bothered, poor HRQoL). Three dimensions are assessed: symptoms, emotions, function. (Lee, N., Keum, Chung, & Lee, 2016; Pluta, 2010)

3.1.3. Short Form Health Survey
The tool is originally constructed for use in the Medical Outcomes Study and not specific to skin. It evaluates 8 dimensions of HRQoL,

including physical functioning, role physical, role emotional, bodily pain, social functioning, general health, vitality, and mental health. The scores range from 0 (poor HRQoL) to 100 (high HRQoL). (Ware & Sherbourne, 1992)

3.1.4. Pediatric Quality of Life Inventory Parent and Child Versions

The tool is used in many disorders and not specific to skin. Evaluates physical function, psychological function, and social function. The scores range from 0 (poor HRQoL) to 100 (high HRQoL). (Varni, Seid, & Rode, 1999)

3.2. Alopecia Areata Specific QOL Instruments

3.2.1. Alopecia Areata Quality of Life Index (AA-QLI)

The AA-QLI was developed from interviews with 50 patients with alopecia areata and clinical expert opinion. A detailed description of the item reduction process is lacking. It shows a good convergent validity against the DLQI. No reliability test has been performed. (Fabbrocini et al., 2013)

3.2.2. Alopecia Areata Quality of Life (AAQ)

The items of the AAQ were developed based on semi-structured interviews with patients with alopecia areata and clinical expert opinion. The instrument demonstrated a good construct and convergent validity in a sample of 122 patients. A good internal consistency was reported for the restriction of activities and concealment dimensions, but it was poor for adaptation. (Endo, Miyachi, & Arakawa, 2012)

3.2.3. Alopecia Areata Symptom Impact Scale (AASIS)

AASIS has been developed using data from 1400 patients from a national patient registry together with clinical experts' reviews. A good content validity was found through cognitive debriefing with 210 patients with AA. Each of the three domains of the questionnaire showed good or excellent internal consistency. (Mendoza, Osei, & Duvic, 2018)

3.3. Quality of Life in Alopecia Areata Is Comparable to Other Diseases

Studies consistently show that patients with alopecia areata experience poor HRQoL compared with the general population. Loss of hair in patients with alopecia areata negatively impacts QoL and is often associated with loss of self-esteem and psychosocial problems. (Abedini et al., 2018) Patients with alopecia areata demonstrate poorer HRQoL than control patients, with realms such as vitality, mental health, emotion, and social functioning. Pediatric patients and their parents also reported to have poorer HRQoL. (Putterman et al., 2019) The impact of alopecia areata on HRQoL is comparable with other chronic, relapsing skin conditions such as psoriasis and atopic dermatitis. DLQI scores of patients with alopecia areata were 5.3 to 13.54, which is similar to scores for patients with psoriasis (5.83 to 13.4) and atopic dermatitis (7.31 to 10.63). (Karia, De Sousa, Shah, Sonavane, & Bharati, 2015) Worth noting is that patients with alopecia areata do not experience physical symptoms directly related to their disease, whereas patients with atopic dermatitis and psoriasis commonly experience pruritus and sleep disturbance. As a result, the true psychosocial impact of alopecia areata may be even greater and therefore warrants a similar level of attention. (Bilgiç et al., 2014)

The poor QoL in patients with alopecia areata may play a role in the development of psychiatric comorbidities such as depression, generalized anxiety, and obsessive-compulsive disorder. One study found a 39% lifetime prevalence of major depressive disorder and a 39% lifetime prevalence of generalized anxiety disorder in patients with alopecia areata. (Okhovat et al., 2019)

Decreased in QoL and related psychiatric comorbidities may be related to feelings of hopelessness, and the relapsing and often progressive course of the condition, creating persistent anxiety about possible future hair loss. Patients experience significant negative effects on social and emotional well-being and mental health. Alopecia areata is not only cosmetic but rather is a medical condition with profound negative health consequences.

CONCLUSION

Alopecia areata is a chronic immune-mediated inflammatory disease of the hair follicle and typically leads to nonscarring hair loss. (Hon KL, 2011) Spontaneous regrowth occurs in many patients with alopecia areata. Around 50% of those with limited patchy hair loss will recover within a year. Hair loss may persist for several years and in some cases the bald patches never regrow. (Tosti, Bellavista, & Iorizzo, 2006)

Clinical factors associated with poor prognosis and high likelihood of relapse include onset in childhood, severe disease (especially alopecia totalis or alopecia universalis), persistence of disease more than one year, band-like involvement of the peripheral temporal and occipital scalp (ophiasis), nail involvement, atopy and family history of alopecia areata. (Alkhalifah, Alsantali, Wang, Mcelwee, & Shapiro, 2010a; Hon KL, 2011; Strazzulla et al., 2018)

Treatment of alopecia areata is highly individualized. The management plan is a shared decision with the patients or their parents and involves careful consideration of the patient's goal of treatment and the benefits and risks of treatment. (Messenger et al., 2012)

REFERENCES

Abedini, R., Hallaji, Z., Lajevardi, V., Nasimi, M., Karimi Khaledi, M., & Tohidinik, H. R. (2018). Quality of life in mild and severe alopecia areata patients. *International Journal of Women's Dermatology,* 4(2), 91-94. doi:10.1016/j.ijwd.2017.07.001.

Alabdulkareem, A. S., Abahussein, A. A., & Okoro, A. (1998). Severe alopecia areata treated with systemic corticosteroids. *International Journal of Dermatology,* 37(8), 622-624. doi:10.1046/j.1365-4362.1998.00422.x.

Alkhalifah, A., Alsantali, A., Wang, E., Mcelwee, K. J., & Shapiro, J. (2010a). Alopecia areata update: Part I. clinical picture, histopathology, and pathogenesis. *Journal of the American Academy of Dermatology,* 62(2), 177-188. doi:10.1016/j.jaad.2009.10.032.

Alkhalifah, A., Alsantali, A., Wang, E., Mcelwee, K. J., & Shapiro, J. (2010b). Alopecia areata update: Part II. treatment. *Journal of the American Academy of Dermatology,* 62(2), 191-202. doi:10.1016/j.jaad.2009.10.031.

Alsantali, A. (2011). Alopecia areata: A new treatment plan. *Clinical, Cosmetic and Investigational Dermatology,* 4, 107-115. doi:10.2147/CCID.S22767.

Bilgiç, Ö, Bilgiç, A., Bahalı, K., Bahali, A. G., Gürkan, A., & Yılmaz, S. (2014). Psychiatric symptomatology and health-related quality of life in children and adolescents with alopecia areata. *Journal of the European Academy of Dermatology and Venereology,* 28(11), 1463-1468. doi:10.1111/jdv.12315.

Bokhari, L., & Sinclair, R. (2018). Treatment of alopecia universalis with topical janus kinase inhibitors – a double blind, placebo, and active controlled pilot study. *International Journal of Dermatology,* 57(12), 1464-1470. doi:10.1111/ijd.14192.

Byun, J. W., Moon, J. H., Bang, C. Y., Shin, J., & Choi, G. S. (2015). Effectiveness of 308-nm excimer laser therapy in treating alopecia areata, determined by examining the treated sides of selected alopecic patches. *Dermatology,* 231(1), 70-76. doi:10.1159/000381912.

Castelo-Soccio, L. (2017). Experience with oral tofacitinib in 8 adolescent patients with alopecia universalis. *Journal of the American Academy of Dermatology,* 76(4), 754-755. doi:10.1016/j.jaad.2016.11.038.

Charuwichitratana, S., Wattanakrai, P., & Tanrattanakorn, S. (2000). Randomized double-blind placebo-controlled trial in the treatment of alopecia areata with 0.25% desoximetasone cream. *Archives of Dermatology,* 136(10), 1276-1277. doi:10.1001/archderm.136.10.1276.

Choe, S. J., Lee, S., Lee, H., Choi, J., & Lee, W. (2018). Efficacy of topical diphenylcyclopropenone maintenance treatment for patients with alopecia areata: A retrospective study. *Journal of the American*

Academy of Dermatology, 78(1), 205-207.e1. doi:10.1016/j.jaad. 2017.07.028.

Choe, S. J., Lee, S., Pi, L. Q., Keum, D. I., Lee, C. H., Kim, B. J., & Lee, W. (2018). Subclinical sensitization with diphenylcyclopropenone is sufficient for the treatment of alopecia areata: Retrospective analysis of 159 cases. *Journal of the American Academy of Dermatology,* 78(3), 515-521.e4. doi:10.1016/j.jaad.2017.10.042.

Coronel-Pérez, I., Rodríguez-Rey, E., & Camacho-Martínez, F. (2010). Latanoprost in the treatment of eyelash alopecia in alopecia areata universalis. *Journal of the European Academy of Dermatology and Venereology,* 24(4), 481-485. doi:10.1111/j.1468-3083.2009.03543.x.

Craiglow, B. G., & King, B. A. (2014). Killing two birds with one stone: Oral tofacitinib reverses alopecia universalis in a patient with plaque psoriasis. *Journal of Investigative Dermatology,* 134(12), 2988-2990. doi:10.1038/jid.2014.260.

Craiglow, B. G., & King, B. A. (2019). Tofacitinib for the treatment of alopecia areata in preadolescent children. *Journal of the American Academy of Dermatology,* 80(2), 568-570. doi:10.1016/j.jaad.2018. 08.041.

Craiglow, B. G., Tavares, D., & King, B. A. (2016). Topical ruxolitinib for the treatment of alopecia universalis. (report). *JAMA Dermatology,* 152(4), 490. doi:10.1001/jamadermatol.2015.4445.

Endo, Y., Miyachi, Y., & Arakawa, A. (2012). Development of a disease-specific instrument to measure quality of life in patients with alopecia areata. *European Journal of Dermatology*, 22(4), 531-536..

Fabbrocini, G., Panariello, L., De Vita, V., Vincenzi, C., Lauro, C., Nappo, D., ... Tosti, A. (2013). Quality of life in alopecia areata: A disease-specific questionnaire. *Journal of the European Academy of Dermatology and Venereology,* 27(3), e276-e281. doi:10.1111/j.1468-3083.2012.04629.x.

Fiedler-Weiss, V. (1987). Topical minoxidil solution (1% and 5%) in the treatment of alopecia areata. *Journal of the American Academy of Dermatology,* 16(3), 745-748. doi:10.1016/S0190-9622(87)80003-8.

Finlay, A. Y., & Khan, G. K. (1994). Dermatology life quality index (DLQI)—a simple practical measure for routine clinical use. *Clinical and Experimental Dermatology,* 19(3), 210-216. doi:10.1111/j.1365-2230.1994.tb01167.x.

Gilhar, A., Keren, A., & Paus, R. (2019). JAK inhibitors and alopecia areata. *The Lancet,* 393(10169), 318-319. doi:10.1016/S0140-6736(18)32987-8.

Gilhar, A., Paus, R., & Kalish, R. S. (2007). Lymphocytes, neuropeptides, and genes involved in alopecia areata. (science in medicine)(clinical report). *Journal of Clinical Investigation,* 117(8), 2019. doi:10.1172/JCI31942.

Healy, E., & Rogers, S. (1993). PUVA treatment for alopecia areata—does it work? A retrospective review of 102 cases. *British Journal of Dermatology,* 129(1), 42-44. doi:10.1111/j.1365-2133.1993.tb03309.x.

Hon K.L., Leung, A.K. (2008). Unusual loss of body hair in childhood: Trichotillomania or alopecia. *Advances in Therapy,* 25(4), 380-387.

Hon, K.L., Leung, A.K. (2011). Alopecia areata. *Recent Patents on Inflammation & Allergy Drug Discovery,* 5(2), 98-107.

Ibrahim, O., Bayart, C. B., Hogan, S., Piliang, M., & Bergfeld, W. F. (2017). Treatment of alopecia areata with tofacitinib. *JAMA Dermatology,* 153(6), 600-602. doi:10.1001/jamadermatol.2017.0001.

Kar, B. R., Handa, S., Dogra, S., & Kumar, B. (2005). Placebo-controlled oral pulse prednisolone therapy in alopecia areata. *Journal of the American Academy of Dermatology,* 52(2), 287-290. doi:10.1016/j.jaad.2004.10.873.

Karia, S., De Sousa, A., Shah, N., Sonavane, S., & Bharati, A. (2015). Psychiatric morbidity and quality of life in skin diseases: A comparison of alopecia areata and psoriasis. *Industrial Psychiatry Journal,* 24(2) doi:10.4103/0972-6748.181724.

Kassim, J. M., Shipman, A. R., Szczecinska, W., Siah, T. W., Lam, M., Chalmers, J., & Macbeth, A. E. (2014). How effective is intralesional injection of triamcinolone acetonide compared with topical treatments in inducing and maintaining hair growth in patients with alopecia areata? A critically appraised topic. *British Journal of Dermatology,* 170(4), 766-771. doi:10.1111/bjd.12863.

Kasumagic-Halilovic, E., & Prohic, A. (2009). Nail changes in alopecia areata: Frequency and clinical presentation. *Journal of the European Academy of Dermatology and Venereology,* 23(2), 240-241. doi:10.1111/j.1468-3083.2008.02830.x.

Kim, B. J., Uk Min, S., Park, K. Y., Choi, J. W., Park, S. W., Youn, S. W., ... Huh, C. H. (2008). Combination therapy of cyclosporine and methylprednisolone on severe alopecia areata. *Journal of Dermatological Treatment,* 19(4), 216-220. doi:10.1080/09546630701846095.

Kuldeep, C., Singhal, H., Khare, A., Mittal, A., Gupta, L., & Garg, A. (2011). Randomized comparison of topical betamethasone valerate foam, intralesional triamcinolone acetonide and tacrolimus ointment in management of localized alopecia areata. *International Journal of Trichology,* 3(1), 20-24. doi:10.4103/0974-7753.82123.

Lee, H. H., Gwillim, E., Patel, K. R., Hua, T., Rastogi, S., Ibler, E., & Silverberg, J. I. (2019). Epidemiology of alopecia areata, ophiasis, totalis and universalis: A systematic review and meta-analysis. *Journal of the American Academy of Dermatology,* doi:10.1016/j.jaad.2019.08.032.

Lee, N., Keum, D. I., Chung, H. C., & Lee, W. (2016). Comparison of quality of life using hair-specific skindex-29 between androgenetic alopecia and alopecia areata. *Journal of the American Academy of Dermatology,* 74(5), AB134-AB134. doi:10.1016/j.jaad.2016.02.527.

Lee, S., Kim, B. J., Lee, Y. B., & Lee, W. (2018). Hair regrowth outcomes of contact immunotherapy for patients with alopecia areata: A systematic review and meta-analysis. *JAMA Dermatology,* 154(10), 1145. doi:10.1001/jamadermatol.2018.2312.

Lenane, P., Macarthur, C., Parkin, P. C., Krafchik, B., DeGroot, J., Khambalia, A., & Pope, E. (2014). Clobetasol propionate, 0.05%, vs hydrocortisone, 1%, for alopecia areata in children: A randomized clinical trial. (clinical report). *JAMA Dermatology,* 150(1), 47. doi:10.1001/jamadermatol.2013.5764.

Leung, A. K., & Robson, W. L. (1993). Hair loss in children. *Journal of the Royal Society of Health*, 113(5), 252-256.

Leung, A. K., Adams, S. P., & Wong, A. H. (2012). Alopecia areata. *Consultant for Pediatricians*, (11), 83-84.

Leung, A. K. C., & Barankin, B. (2015). Congenital triangular alopecia - report of a case and review of the literature. *Aperito Journal of Dermatology*, 2(2), 112.

Leung, A. K. C., & Barankin, B. (2016). Incidence of congenital triangular alopecia. *Anais Brasileiros De Dermatologia*, 91(4), 556. doi:10.1590/abd1806-4841.20165431.

Leung, A, K. C., Barankin, B., & Leong, K. F. (2018). An 8-Year-Old Child with Delayed Diagnosis of Netherton Syndrome. *Case Reports in Pediatrics*. doi:10.1155/2018/9434916.

Leung, A. K., Leong, K. F., & Barankin, B. (2019). Trachyonychia. *The Journal of Pediatrics*. pii: S0022-3476(19)31092-3. doi: 10.1016/j.jpeds.2019.08.034.

Liu, L. Y., Craiglow, B. G., Dai, F., & King, B. A. (2017). Tofacitinib for the treatment of severe alopecia areata and variants: A study of 90 patients. *Journal of the American Academy of Dermatology*, 76(1), 22-28. doi:10.1016/j.jaad.2016.09.007.

Liu, L. Y., Craiglow, B. G., & King, B. A. (2018). Tofacitinib 2% ointment, a topical janus kinase inhibitor, for the treatment of alopecia areata: A pilot study of 10 patients. *Journal of the American Academy of Dermatology*, 78(2), 403-404.e1. doi:10.1016/j.jaad.2017.10.043.

Liu, L. Y., & King, B. A. (2019). Ruxolitinib for the treatment of severe alopecia areata. *Journal of the American Academy of Dermatology*, 80(2), 566-568. doi:10.1016/j.jaad.2018.08.040.

Liu, L. Y., King, B. A., & Craiglow, B. G. (2016). Health-related quality of life (HRQoL) among patients with alopecia areata (AA): A systematic review. *Journal of the American Academy of Dermatology*, 75(4), 806-812.e3. doi:10.1016/j.jaad.2016.04.035.

Lu, W., Shapiro, J., Yu, M., Barekatain, A., Lo, B., Finner, A., & McElwee, K. (2006). Alopecia areata: Pathogenesis and potential for therapy. *Expert Reviews in Molecular Medicine,* 8(14), 1-19. doi:10.1017/S146239940601101X.

Lucky, A. W., Piacquadio, D. J., Ditre, C. M., Dunlap, F., Kantor, I., Pandya, A. G., ... Tharp, M. D. (2004). A randomized, placebo-controlled trial of 5% and 2% topical minoxidil solutions in the treatment of female pattern hair loss. *Journal of the American Academy of Dermatology,* 50(4), 541-553. doi:10.1016/j.jaad.2003.06.014.

Mackay-Wiggan, J., Jabbari, A., Nguyen, N., Cerise, J. E., Clark, C., Ulerio, G., ... Clynes, R. (2016). Oral ruxolitinib induces hair regrowth in patients with moderate-to-severe alopecia areata. *JCI Insight,* 1(15), e89790. doi:10.1172/jci.insight.89790.

Mendoza, T. R., Osei, J., & Duvic, M. (2018). The utility and validity of the alopecia areata symptom impact scale in measuring disease-related symptoms and their effect on functioning. *The Journal of Investigative Dermatology. Symposium Proceedings,* 19(1), S41. doi:10.1016/j.jisp.2017.10.009.

Messenger, A. G., Mckillop, J., Farrant, P., Mcdonagh, A. J., & Sladden, M. (2012). British association of dermatologists' guidelines for the management of alopecia areata 2012. *British Journal of Dermatology,* 166(5), 916-926. doi:10.1111/j.1365-2133.2012.10955.x.

Mitchell, A. J., & Krull, E. A. (1984). Alopecia areata: Pathogenesis and treatment. *Journal of the American Academy of Dermatology,* 11(5), 763. doi:10.1016/S0190-9622(84)80450-8.

Miteva, M., & Tosti, A. (2012). Hair and scalp dermatoscopy. *Journal of the American Academy of Dermatology,* 67(5), 1040-1048. doi:10.1016/j.jaad.2012.02.013.

Okhovat, J., Grogan, T., Duan, L., & Goh, C. (2017). Willingness to pay and quality of life in alopecia areata. *Journal of the American Academy of Dermatology,* 77(6), 1183-1184. doi:10.1016/j.jaad.2017.07.023.

Okhovat, J., Marks, D. H., Manatis-Lornell, A., Hagigeorges, D., Locascio, J. J., & Senna, M. M. (2019). Association between alopecia areata, anxiety, and depression: A systematic review and meta-analysis.

Journal of the American Academy of Dermatology, doi:10.1016/j.jaad. 2019.05.086.

Olsen, E. A., Carson, S. C., & Turney, E. A. (1992). Systemic steroids with or without 2% topical minoxidil in the treatment of alopecia areata. *Archives of Dermatology,* 128(11), 1467-1473. doi:10.1001/archderm. 1992.01680210045005.

Park, H., Kim, M., Lee, J. S., Yoon, H., Huh, C., Kwon, O., & Cho, S. (2017). Oral tofacitinib monotherapy in korean patients with refractory moderate-to-severe alopecia areata: A case series. *Journal of the American Academy of Dermatology,* 77(5), 978-980. doi:10.1016/ j.jaad.2017.06.027.

Paus, R., Nickoloff, B. J., & Ito, T. (2005). A 'hairy' privilege. *Trends in Immunology,* 26(1), 32. doi:10.1016/j.it.2004.09.014.

Phan, K., Ramachandran, V., & Sebaratnam, D. F. (2019). Methotrexate for alopecia areata: A systematic review and meta-analysis. *Journal of the American Academy of Dermatology,* 80(1), 120-127.e2. doi:10.1016/j.jaad.2018.06.064.

Pluta, R. (2010). Development and validation of skindex-teen, a quality-of-life instrument for adolescents with skin disease. *Jama,* 304(16), 1768..

Porter, D., & Burton, J. L. (1971). A comparison of intra-lesional triaminolone hexa-cetonide and triamcinolone acetonide in alopecia areata. *British Journal of Dermatology,* 85(3), 272-273. doi:10.1111/j. 1365-2133.1971.tb07230.x.

Price, V. H. (1987). Double-blind, placebo-controlled evaluation of topical minoxidil in extensive alopecia areata. *Journal of the American Academy of Dermatology,* 16(3), 730-736. doi:10.1016/S0190-9622 (87)70095-4.

Putterman, E., & Castelo-Soccio, L. (2018). Topical 2% tofacitinib for children with alopecia areata, alopecia totalis, and alopecia universalis. *Journal of the American Academy of Dermatology,* 78(6), 1207-1209.e1. doi:10.1016/j.jaad.2018.02.031.

Putterman, E., Patel, D. P., Andrade, G., Harfmann, K. L., Hogeling, M., Cheng, C. E., ... Castelo-Soccio, L. (2019). *Severity of disease and quality of life in parents of children with alopecia areata, totalis, and universalis:* A prospective, cross-sectional study doi:10. 1016/j.jaad.2018.12.051.

Rencz, F., Gulácsi, L., Péntek, M., Wikonkál, N., Baji, P., & Brodszky, V. (2016). Alopecia areata and health-related quality of life: A systematic review and meta-analysis. *British Journal of Dermatology,* 175(3), 561-571. doi:10.1111/bjd.14497.

Rokhsar, C. K., Shupack, J. L., Vafai*, J. J., & Washenik, K. (1998). Efficacy of topical sensitizers in the treatment of alopecia areata. *Journal of the American Academy of Dermatology,* 39(5), 751-761. doi:10.1016/S0190-9622(98)70048-9.

Roseborough, I., Lee, H., Chwalek, J., Stamper, R. L., & Price, V. H. (2009). Lack of efficacy of topical latanoprost and bimatoprost ophthalmic solutions in promoting eyelash growth in patients with alopecia areata. *Journal of the American Academy of Dermatology,* 60(4), 705. doi:10.1016/j.jaad.2008.08.029.

Ross, E. K., Bolduc, C., Lui, H., & Shapiro, J. (2005). Lack of efficacy of topical latanoprost in the treatment of eyebrow alopecia areata. *Journal of the American Academy of Dermatology,* 53(6), 1095. doi:10.1016/ j.jaad.2005.06.031.

Strazzulla, L. C., Wang, E. H. C., Avila, L., Lo Sicco, K., Brinster, N., Christiano, A. M., & Shapiro, J. (2018). Alopecia areata: Disease characteristics, clinical evaluation, and new perspectives on pathogenesis: Disease characteristics, clinical evaluation, and new perspectives on pathogenesis. *Journal of the American Academy of Dermatology,* 78(1), 1-12. doi:10.1016/j.jaad.2017.04.1141.

Taylor, C. R., & Hawk, J. L. M. (1995). PUVA treatment of alopecia areata partialis, totalis and universalis: Audit of 10 years' experience at st john's institute of dermatology. *British Journal of Dermatology,* 133(6), 914-918. doi:10.1111/j.1365-2133.1995.tb06925.x.

Tosti, A., Bellavista, S., & Iorizzo, M. (2006). Alopecia areata: A long term follow-up study of 191 patients. *Journal of the American Academy of Dermatology,* 55(3), 438-441. doi:10.1016/ j.jaad.2006.05.008.

Trink, A., Sorbellini, E., Bezzola, P., Rodella, L., Rezzani, R., Ramot, Y., & Rinaldi, F. (2013). A randomized, double-blind, placebo- and active-controlled, half-head study to evaluate the effects of platelet-rich plasma on alopecia areata. *British Journal of Dermatology,* 169(3), 690-694. doi:10.1111/bjd.12397.

Valenzuela, F., Korman, N. J., Bissonnette, R., Bakos, N., Tsai, T. -., Harper, M. K., ... Gardner, A. C. (2018). Tofacitinib in patients with moderate-to-severe chronic plaque psoriasis: Long-term safety and efficacy in an open-label extension study. (report). *British Journal of Dermatology,* 179(4), 853. doi:10.1111/bjd.16798.

Vañó-Galván, S., Hermosa-Gelbard, Á, Sánchez-Neila, N., Miguel-Gómez, L., Saceda-Corralo, D., Rodrigues-Barata, R., ... Jaén, P. (2016). Pulse corticosteroid therapy with oral dexamethasone for the treatment of adult alopecia totalis and universalis. *Journal of the American Academy of Dermatology,* 74(5), 1005-1007. doi:10.1016/j.jaad.2015.12.026.

Varni, W., J., Seid, A., M., & Rode, A., C. (1999). The PedsQL™: Measurement model for the pediatric quality of life inventory. *Medical Care,* 37(2), 126-139. doi:10.1097/00005650-199902000-00003.

Villasante Fricke, A.,C., & Miteva, M. (2015). Epidemiology and burden of alopecia areata: A systematic review. *Clinical, Cosmetic and Investigational Dermatology,* 8, 397. doi:10.2147/CCID.S53985.

Ware, John E., & Sherbourne, C. D. (1992). The MOS 36-item short-form health survey (SF-36): I. conceptual framework and item selection. *Medical Care,* 30(6), 473-483..

Wasyłyszyn, T., Kozłowski, W., & Zabielski, S. (2007). Changes in distribution pattern of CD8 lymphocytes in the scalp in alopecia areata during treatment with diphencyprone. *Archives of Dermatological Research,* 299(5-6), 231-237. doi:10.1007/s00403-007-0759-4.

Whiting, D. A. (2003). Histopathologic features of alopecia areata: A new look. *Archives of Dermatology,* 139(12), 1555-1559. doi:10.1001/archderm.139.12.1555.

Wiseman, M. C., Shapiro, J., Macdonald, N., & Lui, H. (2001). Predictive model for immunotherapy of alopecia areata with diphencyprone. *Archives of Dermatology,* 137(8), 1063-1068.

Wollenhaupt, J., Silverfield, J., Lee, E. B., Curtis, J. R., Wood, S. P., Soma, K., ... Riese, R. J. (2014). Safety and efficacy of tofacitinib, an oral janus kinase inhibitor, for the treatment of rheumatoid arthritis in open-label, longterm extension studies. *The Journal of Rheumatology,* 41(5), 837. doi:10.3899/jrheum.130683.

Xing, L., Dai, Z., Jabbari, A., Jane, E. C., Claire, A. H., Gong, W., ... Clynes, R. (2014). Alopecia areata is driven by cytotoxic T lymphocytes and is reversed by JAK inhibition. *Nature Medicine,* 20(9) doi:10.1038/nm.3645.

Yeo, I. K., Ko, E. J., No, Y. A., Lim, E. S., Park, K. Y., Li, K., ... Hong, C. K. (2015). Comparison of high-dose corticosteroid pulse therapy and combination therapy using oral cyclosporine with low-dose corticosteroid in severe alopecia areata. *Annals of Dermatology*, 27(6), 676. doi:10.5021/ad.2015.27.6.676.

Zakaria, W., Passeron, T., Ostovari, N., Lacour, J., & Ortonne, J. (2004). 308-nm excimer laser therapy in alopecia areata. *Journal of the American Academy of Dermatology,* 51(5), 837-838. doi:10.1016/j.jaad.2004.05.026.

Zhao, Y., & Zhang, R. (2018). Congenital triangular alopecia: A brief report. (letters to editor)(letter to the editor). *International Journal of Trichology,* 10(6), 290. doi:10.4103/ijt.ijt_68_18.

In: Alopecia
Editor: Pietro Gentile
ISBN: 978-1-53617-008-5
© 2020 Nova Science Publishers, Inc.

Chapter 4

A UNIQUE COCKTAIL OF REGENERATIVE TRICHOLOGY POWERED WITH RIGHT NUTRITION-A NOVEL APPROACH TO ADDRESS HAIR DISORDERS

Suruchi Garg and Bhumika Chowdhary
Department of Aesthetics, Regenerative and
Intervention Dermatology, Aura Skin Institute,
Chandigarh, India

ABSTRACT

Hair disorders and their treatments are one of the most intriguing and challenging areas in dermatology practice. Modern dermatology, trichology and regenerative surgery is more result oriented. It aims at restoring the lost hair volume through mesotherapy and platelet rich plasma therapy, or transplanting hormone insensitive -permanent follicular units to introduce new follicles in place of dormant and dead follicles through hair transplant surgery. Considering the huge impact of environmental triggers, like faulty lifestyle and aberrant eating habits, the treatment of hair disorders may not be holistic, unless underlying nutritional deficiencies are corrected. Hair is a neuroendocrine organ; hormone and neuromediator production is in similar lines to that produced by brain, especially in conditions of oxidative and psycho-emotional stress, ultraviolet irradiation, nutritional and sensory stimuli and microbial signals. A sound knowledge in the pathogenesis and diagnosis of hair disorders, correction of underlying nutritional deficiencies and psycho-emotional triggers along with substantial medical treatment is the core approach to the treatment of hair disorders. Regenerative and intervention trichology is a promising, result oriented and ever evolving field in treatment of difficult to treat hair disorders.

INTRODUCTION

Hair disorders and their treatments are one of the most intriguing and challenging areas in dermatology practice. The conventional dermatology deals with the correct diagnosis of underlying cause to the concerned problem and regaining hair growth with the recommended medications. Modern dermatology, trichology and regenerative surgery on the other hand, is more result oriented. It aims at restoring the lost hair volume through mesotherapy and platelet rich plasma therapy, or transplanting hormone insensitive -permanent follicular units to introduce new follicles in place of dormant and dead follicles through hair transplant surgery (Garg 2016). Considering the huge impact of environmental triggers like faulty lifestyle and aberrant eating habits, the treatment of hair disorders may not be holistic unless the underlying contributing nutritional deficiencies are properly diagnosed and treated as per recommendations (Garg and Sangwan 2019).

IMPACT OF PROBLEM

Hair loss leads to adverse psychology including low confidence and negative influence on social interactions as depicted by a study, wherein 52% women and 28% men being extremely upset with hair loss (Cash 1999). Current lifestyle and stressful job profiles are the environmental triggers which are contributing viciously and are creating an epidemic like situation in hair disorders as encountered frequently in dermatology and trichology practice(Garg and Sangwan 2019; Gan 2005).

CLASSIFICATION OF ACQUIRED HAIR DISORDERS

1. Non-Scarring Alopecias

(i) Patterned hair loss
(ii) Alopecia areata
(iii) Telogen effluvium: acute/chronic/dug induced

2. Scarring Alopecias

(i) Congenital: epidermal naevi, aplasia cutis, Incontinentia pigmenti, Epidermolysis bullosa
(ii) Infections
    (a) Bacterial: folliculitis, furuncle, carbuncle
    (b) Fungal: Kerion, favus, rarely Tinea capitis
    (c) Viral: herpes zoster, varicella
    (d) Parasitic: Leishmaniasis, Treponema: Syphilis
(iii) Inflammation: Folliculitis decalvans, Dissecting cellulitis, Acne keloidalis nuchae, Discoid lupus erythematosus, Lichen planus pigmentosus and its variants (Classic, Frontal fibrosing alopecia, Graham-Little-Piccardi-Lassueur syndrome), Central centrifugal cicatricial alopecia, Acne necrotica, autoimmune blistering disorders
(iv) Sclerosing disorders: Morphea, Lichen sclerosus, Scleroderma, Sclerodermoid porphyria cutanea tarda, graft versus host disease.
(v) Granulomatous disorders: Sarcoidosis, Necrobiosis lipoidica
(vi) Traumatic: Mechanical, burns, dermatitis artefacta, traction alopecia, radiation dermatitis

(vii) Neoplastic
   (a) Benign: benign adnexal tumours
   (b) Malignant:
       Primary – cutaneous T cell lymphoma, SCC, BCC
       Secondary – metastasis from other sites

APPROACH TO A PATIENT OF HAIR FALL

A detailed history pertaining to hair fall, whether it is rapid in onset or chronic, diffuse or localized, any associated symptoms like, itching, burning or pain; immediate past history of disease, drug intake, trauma or stress, seasonal variation, history of similar episodes in family should be evaluated. A detailed dietary history with regard to timings, quantity and quality of meals should be undertaken with special emphasis on prolonged overnight starvation or crash dieting in recent past as it may trigger autophagy in skin and hair tissues. A recent study mentions that in state of regular prolonged starvation or low protein intake, body has preferential diversion of proteins and micronutrients towards metabolically more active tissues like muscle (Garg and Sangwan 2019). The important functions like tissue repair, immunity, antibody production, enzymatic activities which are primarily handled by proteins are given preference over relatively not so essential high primarily protein based structures like skin and hair (Garg and Sangwan 2019). In fact, another concept is to break down these protein rich tissues to derive and divert nutrients for functionally more vital areas. So to say, body is in autophagy or self-eating mode when total protein intake is less than half of what is recommended for a particular body type based on weight and physical activity (Garg and Sangwan 2019).

A thorough clinical examination of hair loss site, size, surface, scarring/non-scarring, discoloration, redness, follicular plugging and condition of perilesional hair should be performed. Hair pull test followed by trichogram may be done by epilating 20- 50 hairs with rubber-shod artery clamp and subsequently analysing under a microscope. The hair root in each growth phase can be counted and examined. More than 20% hair in telogen phase indicates increased hair shedding (Whiting 1996). On the other hand non-invasive trichoscan aids in reaching anagen to telogen ratio but are not helpful in picking up disorders of hair root (Hoffmann 2008). Presently high resolution video-dermoscopy helps in picking up useful signs like broom sign, tulip sign, exclamation sign, flame signs to diagnose different disorders with ease (Tosti 2007). Besides picking up the density, diameter and skin texture, it helps the clinician in diagnosis of underlying cause without letting the patient undergo invasive procedure of skin biopsy. Last but not the least; skin biopsy is the gold standard diagnostic investigation for a conclusive diagnosis specially to rule out the disease process in scarring alopecias.

Hair is considered to be a neuroendocrine organ studded with nerves, blood vessels, hormone receptors for thyroid, vitamin D, melatonin, androgens, etc. and every little change in blood levels of these hormones has an implication on hair health. There is enough evidence to suggest the role of skin and hair as neuro-endocrine organs (Paus 2006). Hormone and neuromediator production here is in similar lines to that produced by brain; especially in conditions of oxidative and psycho-emotional stress, ultraviolet irradiation, nutritional and sensory stimuli and microbial signals; the flow of hormones and their effects in skin and hair tissue is an extrapolation of that expressed in brain (Paus 2010). Thus the endocrine organs, the brain, peripheral nervous system and peripheral tissues like skin and hair work in harmony and interaction of similar cognate receptors in turn maintaining almost same response in periphery (Paus 2006; Paus 2010; Paus 2011; Arck 2006). Authors believe that owing to same ectodermal origin for brain, skin and hair and structurally considering their proteinaceous nature; the excessive stress leading to self-destruction of skin and hair in regular starvation states triggers same autophagy or self-eating signals in brain leading to diseases like Alzheimer's disease and other degenerative disorders (Garg and Sangwan 2019).

When a clinician encounters a patient with hair loss, it is important to consider it as an immediate health concern and there should be a multipronged and methodically treatment approach. Detailed blood tests including complete hemogram, renal and liver function tests, serum vitamin D, B12, zinc levels, iron studies, Thyroid function tests, fasting blood sugar, lipid profile should be performed in all cases; connective tissue work up, hormonal profile or treponemal serology should be advised if relevant after history and clinical examination.

The quality of hair is an indirect reflection of good health and the results in hair disorder depend a lot on the approach of a treating physician and it is highly recommended by authors to address all the underlying deficiencies or deranged results. This approach helps not only in faster resolution of problem but also in reducing the risk of recurrence on withdrawal of therapy; in general applicable for all hair disorders irrespective of underlying cause. A balanced diet rich in proteins, vitamins and minerals, avoiding direct and processed carbohydrates and taking early morning breakfast in accordance with hormonal surge may help in maintaining good results in long run (Garg and Sangwan 2019). Garg et al. conducted a study on 98 patients of skin and hair disorders to understand the co-relation of autophagy and protein intake. Out of a total of 42 patients presenting with different types of alopecias, 90% of Androgenetic alopecia patients were deficient in their protein intake and 55% were found severely deficient consuming less than 30g protein per day. Most of female pattern hair loss patients (90.9%) and three fourth (75%) of telogen effluvium patients were severely deficient. All patients presenting with alopecia areata were severely deficient in protein intake and were also missing their breakfast; possibly triggering deregulated autophagy leading to autoimmune reaction against hair follicles. Interestingly the subjects consuming high carbohydrate- low protein diet showed chronic perifollicular inflammation, besides showing thinning of hair diameter and perifollicular atrophic halos; similar findings were conspicuously absent in subjects consuming recommended protein diet (Garg and Sangwan 2019). There is similar study showing beneficial effects of micronutrients and anti-oxidants, emphasizing their role in countering reactive oxygen species and free radical injuries (Rajput 2010).

TREATMENT APPROACH

1. Non-Scarring Alopecias

Patterned hair loss: It is the most common form of hair loss encountered in males and females and FDA approves only three types of therapies for the treatment; topical minoxidil and low level light therapy for both men and women, and oral finasteride only for men (Blumeyer 2011; Rogers 2008). Minoxidil is associated with its own set of side effects like contact dermatitis (6.5%), hypertrichosis (upto 5%), headache, etc. (Blume-Peytavi 2011; Messenger 2004). Finasteride, on the other hand is more associated with sexual dysfunction and post finasteride syndrome manifesting with psychosis and depression (Mella 2010). Interestingly, more awareness due to the information available on internet is leading many patients aversive to take up these treatment options. Low level light therapy is slow to act and in practice, patients tend to lose patience before they start seeing results.

Women having female pattern hair loss usually suffer from underlying hormonal issues especially polycystic ovarian disease or androgen resistance. The basic cause to this entity has been documented to be high glycaemic food (Spencer 1998). Low levels of ferritin have been documented in female pattern hair loss disorder (Kantor 2003). Usually these patients thrive on food rich in processed carbohydrates and are frequently found to be deficient in vitamins (vitamin D and B12) and essential minerals (iron stores and zinc levels) (Garg and Sangwan 2019).

There are upcoming topical therapies like topical prostaglandin analogues, topical peptides and topical stem cell therapies which are finding their place in restoring hair growth and various case series with positive effect on hair growth are coming up making a place in conjunction with minoxidil or as monotherapy for the treatment of hair loss (Takahashi 2001; Takahashi 2005). Results of topical stem cell therapy in a case of telogen effluvium have been shown in Figure 1.

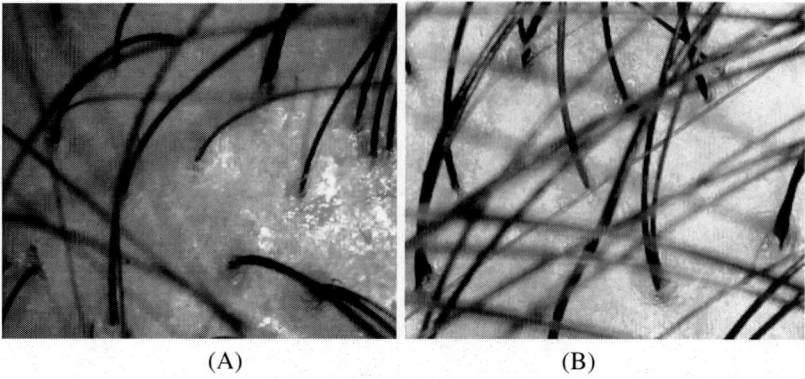

(A) (B)

Figure 1. Baseline image with acute telogen effluvium (terminal- T/intermediate-I:13/4) (A) improvement in hair fall and diameter, 2 months after the use of topical plant based stem cell therapy (T/I:16/2)(B).

More and more studies are available documenting the beneficial role of platelet rich plasma therapy in male and female patterned hair loss. The role is in rejuvenating basement membrane through PDGF, EGF and other growth factors. The mechanism of injury and in turn healing tends to stimulate the epidermal stem cells and also initiate nephronectin- integrin signals over basement membrane, in turn stimulating the bulge portion of stem cells and bulge portion of arrector pili muscle; all three together constitute the "golden anchorage" as depicted in Figure 2. The whole cascade of events, in turn starts migration of stem cells downwards towards dormant papilla, thus letting the hair follicle enter the anagen or growing phase again (Garg 2017; Garg 2018). The results of PRP therapy have been shown in Figure 3 and 4 in patterned hair loss.

More recently, follicular suspension harbouring stem cells have been used as a monotherapy to demonstrate improved hair growth in androgenetic alopecia (Gentile 2019). Another study demonstrates the benefit of combination of permanent zone follicular suspension with platelet rich plasma therapy in improving hair line which was otherwise not attained with PRP as a monotherapy as shown in Figure 5. Follicular suspension might be useful in delivering more permanent signals to otherwise dormant native hair and also activating dormant secondary follicles (Garg and Saginatham 2019).

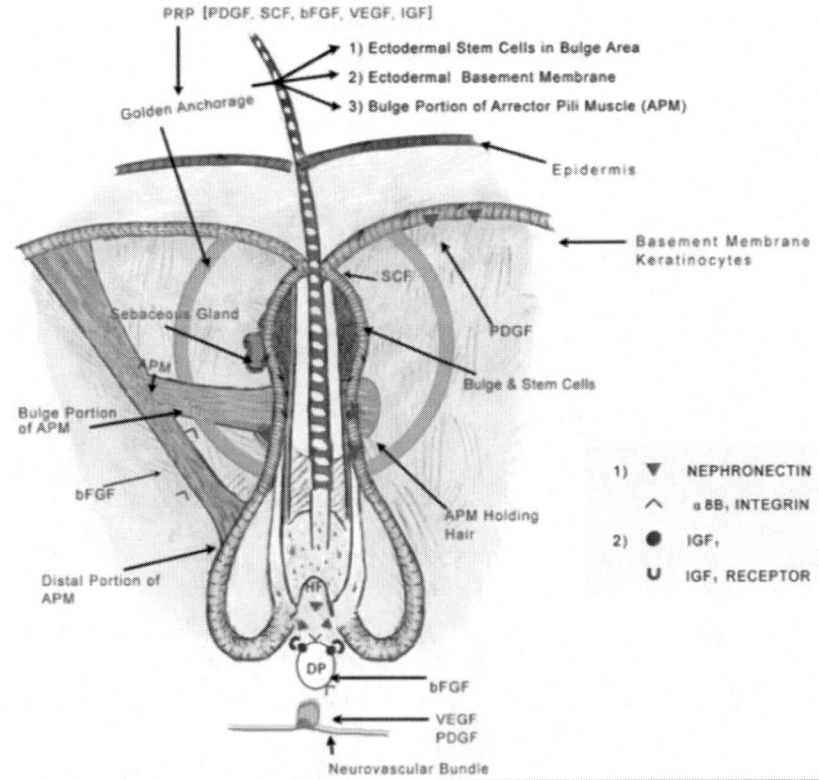

Figure 2. Hair model demonstrating the ' Golden anchorage' comprising of ectodermal basement membrane, stem cells and bulge portion of arector pili muscle, vital in initiating hair growth signals. The figure also highlights the role of various growth factors in rejuvenating different parts of hair follicle unit. (Photo courtesy: Garg S, Manchanda S. Platelet-rich plasma—an 'Elixir' for treatment of alopecia: personal experience on 117 patients with review of literature. Stem Cell Investig 2017; 4: 64).

Hair transplant is a promising option for those who are looking for a more long lasting solution for baldness as the follicular reserve comes from hormone insensitive occipital area or body hair grafts with impressive results. Addition of PRP therapy during transplant enhances graft survival, reduces catagen fall, aids in re-entry of new follicles into anagen phase and activates the dormant hair follicles as depicted in randomized control trial in 40 FUE hair transplant subjects (Garg 2016). The results after 5 months of FUE hair transplant combined with follicular suspension along with

PRP therapy in patient of androgenetic alopecia are shared in Figure 6 by the author. The patient was given only topical 5% minoxidil, peptide based solution and oral multivitamins for 6 months and no oral finasteride was prescribed.

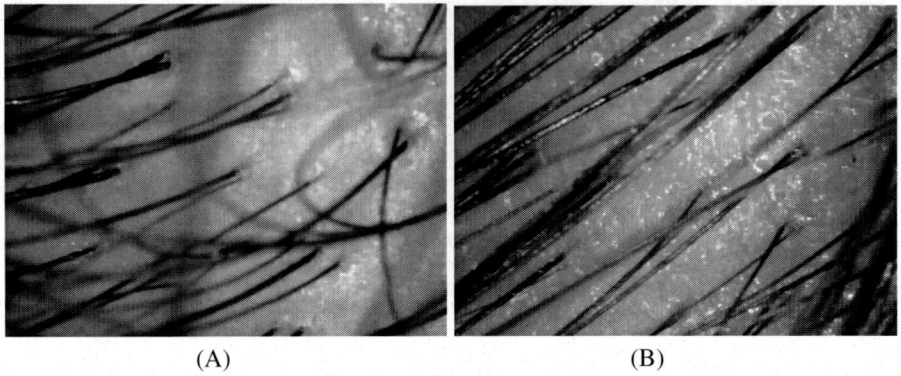

(A) (B)

Figure 3. Androgenetic alopecia along in overlap with telogen effluvium secondary to nutritional deficiency, T/I: 21/7 (A) Improvement in hair diameter, density and skin texture after 3 sessions of PRP therapy, balanced diet and nutritional supplements, T/I:30/4 (B).

Alopecia areata: The standard therapy of minoxidil application and oral supplementation of multivitamins is helpful in some cases of alopecia areata. Intralesional low dose steroid injections or in rare cases oral steroids are useful. In progressive disease immunosuppressants like oral mini pulse therapy work well to halt the autoimmune phenomenon (Luczak 2013; Acikgoz 2014). Other immunosuppressants like weekly methotrexate with or without glucocorticoids or azathioprine may help in resistant cases (Farshi 2010). An Indian study conducted on 50 subjects of alopecia areata demonstrates low serum level of zinc in comparison to controls, in atomic absorption spectroscopy (Bhat 2009). All the underlying deficiencies must be corrected in AA, as these patients are frequently found to be suffering with concomitant hypothyroidism or other autoimmune disorders like vitiligo, lichen planus to name a few (Garg and Sangwan 2019). Topical minoxidil, topical steroids or intralesional steroids are mainstay of therapy in alopecia areata. Simultaneously, topical irritants like squaric acid dibutyl ester (SADBE) or diphencyclopropene (DPCP) can be used as adjuvants to enhance hair growth by inducing delayed type 4 hypersensitivity reaction leading to competitive inhibition of responsible T lymphocytes. A study found squaric acid dibutyl ester superior to topical calcipotriol in alopecia areata, totalis and universalis in a cohort of 28 patients (Orecchia 1995).

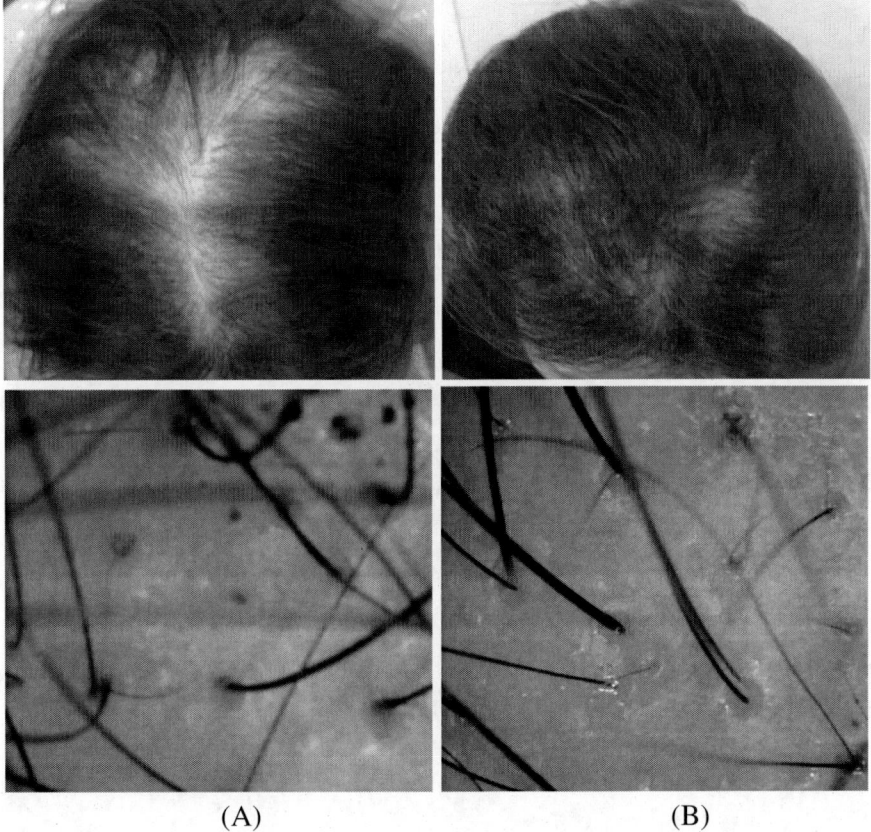

(A)   (B)

Figure 4. Female pattern hair loss with perifollicular atrophic halos, shiny skin texture, closed follicular ostia and miniaturised hair follicles on video microscopy 50x, T/I: 12/5 (A) Improvement in diameter and density, filling up and shrinking of perifollicular halos, improved skin texture and appearance of new hair follicles after 3 sessions of PRP therapy, balanced diet and nutritional supplements T/I: 15/10(B).

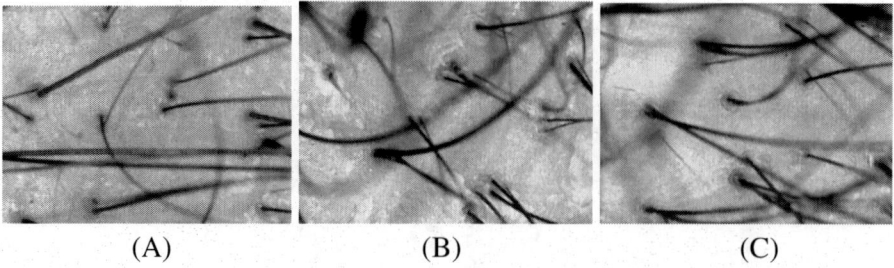

(A) (B) (C)

Figure 5. Androgenetic alopecia T/I: 16/9 (A)1 month after the follicular suspension with platelet rich plasma therapy, noticeable change in hair density, diameter, skin texture and appearance of multiple secondary hair follicles, T/I:22/6 (B) 6 months later, the results are maintained although there is appearance of perifollicular atrophic halo22/5(C).

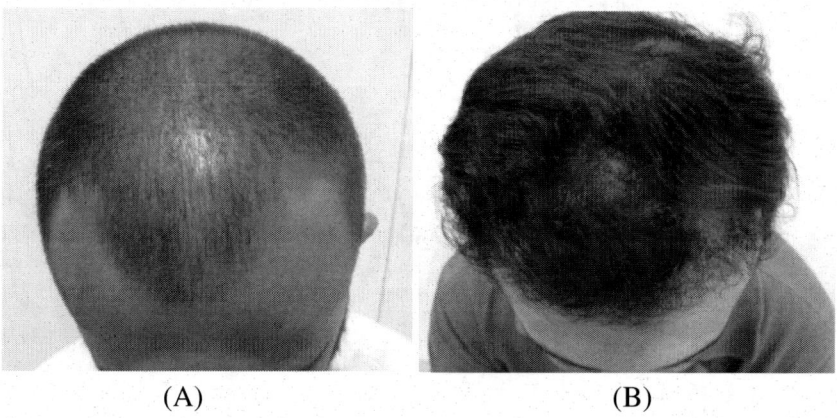

(A) (B)

Figure 6. Androgenetic alopecia (A) 5 months post FUE hair transplant powered with follicular suspension and intra-operative injectable PRP therapy along with balanced diet, topical 5% minoxidil and peptide based solution along with oral multivitamins in follow up period.

The role of platelet rich plasma is beneficial here as PRP therapy starts sending beneficial signals of hair regrowth and start creating a receptive environment by anti-apoptosis and neovascularisation (Singh 2015; Donovan 2015; El Taieb 2017). Chronic patches resistant to these therapies in a stable case of alopecia areata can be considered for hair transplant but chances of recurrence of disease should be explained to the patient (Civas 2010). Interestingly, a transplanted case of androgenetic alopecia later developed patches of alopecia areata but transplanted hair were characteristically spared, possibly explaining hair transplant as more permanent treatment option for resistant AA patients (Yong 2017). Underlying emotional trauma or stress must be dealt with alongside the medical and interventional treatments as it has been implicated as a major trigger in first episode and subsequent recurrences (Manolache 2009).

Telogen effluvium: This is a condition where in numerous hair follicles enter into telogen or the shedding phase leading to excessive hair fall along with roots. The condition can be acute if there is immediate history of disease, culprit drug intake, crash dieting, trauma, stress or harsh salon procedures in past 3-4 months. Usually, the hair regrows in such cases with minimal basic support and once the patient tides over the crisis. On the other hand, chronic telogen effluvium could be secondary to hormonal imbalance or underlying deficient nutritional stores, both conditions viciously inter-related and as explained earlier correction of all the aberrations should be addressed. If uncorrected, it may eventually lead to scarring and progresses to female pattern hair loss. Besides standard medical therapy, platelet rich plasma is useful in strengthening and improving variable hair diameter, captured in video microscopic images as depicted in Figure 7. It helps in flowing more nutrients by improving blood supply through neovascularisation and improving hair cycle length by increasing anagen and shortening the telogen phase (Garg 2017).

2. Scarring Alopecia

Scarring alopecias are difficult to treat hair disorders as these are heterogeneous group of disorders that can destroy the hair follicles irreversibly. An approach through conventional dermatology aids in tackling the underlying cause which could be infectious, inflammatory or autoimmune. Once acute insult is taken care of, the hair follicle reservoir needs to be restored and hair restoration techniques have been dramatically revolutionised to incorporate minute precision (Ekelem 2019). Currently, follicular unit extraction (FUE) is the gold standard technique aiding in harvesting individual hair follicular units without use of sutures and visibly minimally evident scarring (Unger 2008). This can be done by making the scarred area more receptive through platelet rich plasma therapy as it starts rejuvenating the basement membrane, stem cells, arrector pili muscles, vessels and nerves utilizing various growth factors like PDGF, SCF, FGF, VEGF, EGF, EDGF, IGF, etc. (Garg 2017). Platelet Rich Plasma therapy can be undertaken before, during or after the hair transplant to improve the survival of transplanted area. Since blood supply is compromised in scarred tissue, PRP therapy helps in neovascularisation besides revitalizing the overall environment (Saxena 2016). In very thin atrophic tissues like en coupe de sabre, post burn scar where there is paucity of skin and subcutis, small punch grafting can be taken up as first surgery to create a healthy skin tissue and later follicular grafts can be implanted (Garg 2017).

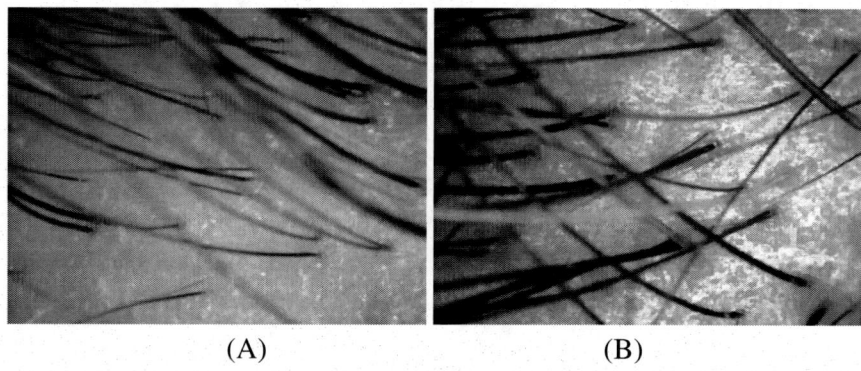

(A) (B)

Figure 7. Chronic telogen effluvium with hypothyroidism, polycystic ovarian disease and diabetes, T/I:18/17(A) after 3 sessions of PRP therapy along with early morning balanced diet rich in proteins, vitamins and minerals T/I:30/7(B).

A case of frontal fibrosing alopecia has been shown to improve with FUE hair transplant with PRP therapy, three years after the disease was stabilized, as shown in Figure 8 (Garg and Pandya 2019). It is recommended for scarring alopecia secondary to underlying inflammatory or autoimmune disease that a disease free period of 2 to 5 years prior to surgery must be observed to reduce chances of reactivation (Ekelem 2019). The future of hair transplant in scarring alopecia is subcutaneous fat transplant before or during the transplant, along with PRP therapy as fat is a reservoir of adipocytes stem cells and nutrition for newly transplanted grafts.

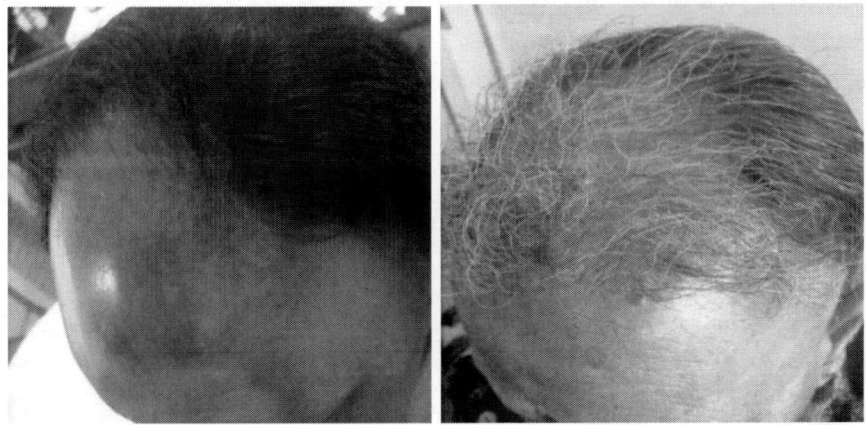

Figure 8. Frontal fibrosing alopecia after 8 months of FUE hair transplant and PRP therapy. He had been following a delayed breakfast and only two meals for past many years. He was advised oral iron supplements to improve ferritin stores, oral vitamin D and B12 supplements in therapeutic doses, topical 2% minoxidil and peptide solutions along with multivitamins in post-operative period. No relapse of disease was seen in two years of follow up period. (Photocourtesy: Garg S, Pandya I, Bhatt S. Follicular Unit Extraction (FUE) Hair Transplantation in Combination with Platelet Rich Plasma for the Treatment of Scarring Alopecia: A Case Series. Archives of Clinical and Medical Case Reports 3 (2019): 299-308.

CONCLUSION

A sound knowledge in the pathogenesis and diagnosis of hair disorders, correction of underlying nutritional deficiencies and psycho-emotional triggers along with substantial medical treatment is the core approach to the treatment of hair disorders. Regenerative and intervention trichology is a promising, result oriented and ever evolving field in treatment of difficult to treat hair disorders.

REFERENCES

Acikgöz, G., Ozmen, I., Cayirli, M., Yeniay, Y. & Kose, O. (2014). Pulse methylprednisolone therapy for the treatment of extensive alopecia areata. *J Dermatolog Treat.*, 25, 164–166.

Arck, P. C., Slominski, A., Theoharides, T. C., Peters, E. M. & Paus, R. (2006). Neuroimmunology of stress: skin takes center stage. *J Invest Dermatol.*, 126, 1697–1704.

Bhat, Y. J., Manzoor, S., Khan, A. R. & Qayooni, S. (2009). Trace element levels in alopecia areata. *Indian J Dermatol Venereol Leprol.*, 75, 29–31.

Blume-Peytavi, U., Hillmann, K., Dietz, E., Canfield, D. & Garcia, B. N. (2011). A randomized, single-blind trial of 5% minoxidil foam once daily versus 2% minoxidil solution twice daily in the treatment of androgenetic alopecia in women. *J Am Acad Dermatol.*, 65, 1126–1134.

Blumeyer, A., Tosti, A., Messenger, A., Reygagne, P., Del Marmol, V., Spuls, P. I., Trakatelli, M., Finner, A., Kiesewetter, F., Trueb, R., Rzany, B. & Blume-Peytavi, U. (2011). Evidence-based (S3) guideline for the treatment of androgenetic alopecia in women and in men. *J Dtsch Dermatol Ges.*, 9, 1–57.

Cash, T. (1999). The psychosocial consequences of androgenetic alopecia: a review of the research literature. *Br J Dermatol.*, 141, 398–405.

Civas, E., Aksoy, B., Aksoy, H. M., Eski, M. & Yucel, K. (2010). Hair transplantation for therapy-resistant alopecia areata of the eyebrows: is it the right choice? *J. Dermatol.*, 37, 823–826.

Donovan, J. (2015). Successful treatment of corticosteroid-resistant ophiasis-type alopecia areata (AA) with platelet-rich plasma (PRP). *JAAD.*, 1, 305-307.

Ekelem, C., Pham, C. & Mesinkovska, N. (2019). A Systematic Review of the Outcome of Hair Transplantation in Primary Scarring Alopecia. *Skin Appendage Disord.*, 5, 65–71.

El Taieb, M. A., Ibrahim, H., Nada, E. A. & Seif Al-Din, M. (2017). Platelets rich plasma versus minoxidil 5% in treatment of alopecia areata: A trichoscopic evaluation. *Dermatol Ther.*, *30*, 1.

Farshi, S., Mansouri, P., Safar, F. & Khiabanloo, S. R. (2010). Could azathioprine be considered as a therapeutic alternative in the treatment of alopecia areata? *A pilot study. Int J Dermatol.*, *49*, 1188–1193.

Gan, D. C. & Sinclair, R. D. (2005). Prevalence of male and female pattern hair loss in Maryborough. *J Investig Dermatol Symp Proc.*, *10*, 184–189.

Garg, S. (2016). Outcome of intra-operative injected platelet-rich plasma therapy during follicular unit extraction hair transplant: A prospective randomised study in forty patients. *J Cutan Aesthet Surg.*, *9*, 157-64

Garg, S. & Manchanda, S. (2017). Platelet-rich plasma—an 'Elixir' for treatment of alopecia: personal experience on 117 patients with review of literature. *Stem Cell Investig.*, *4*, 64.

Garg, S., Manchanda, S. & Garg, C. (2018). The Wonder Tool Platelet Rich Plasma in Cosmetic Dermatology, Trichology and Hair Transplant, Dermatologic Surgery and Procedures, Pierre Vereecken, IntechOpen, DOI: 10.5772/intechopen.70287.

Garg, S., Pandya, I. & Bhatt, S. (2019). Follicular Unit Extraction (FUE) Hair Transplantation in Combination with Platelet Rich Plasma for the Treatment of Scarring Alopecia: A Case Series. *Archives of Clinical and Medical Case Reports.*, *3*, 299-308.

Garg, S., Saginatham, H. & Badheka, A. (2019). Use of Stem Cells in Intervention Dermatology and Trichology: A New Hope. *J Stem Cell Res Dev Ther. S1004.*

Garg, S. & Sangwan, A. (2019). Dietary protein deficit and deregulated autophagy: A new Clinico-diagnostic perspective in pathogenesis of early aging, skin, and hair disorders. *Indian Dermatol Online J.*, *10*, 115-124.

Gentile, P. & Garcovich, S. (2019). Advances in Regenerative Stem Cell Therapy in Androgenic Alopecia and Hair Loss: Wnt Pathway, Growth-Factor, and Mesenchymal Stem Cell Signaling Impact

Analysis on Cell Growth and Hair Follicle Development. *Cells.*, 8, 466.

Hoffmann, R. (2008). TrichoScan, a GCP-validated tool to measure hair growth. *J Eur Acad Dermatol Venereol.*, 22, 132–134.

Kantor, J., Kessler, L. J., Brooks, D. G. & Cotsarelis, G. (2003). Decreased serum ferritin is associated with alopecia in women. *J Invest Dermatol.*, 121, 985–988.

Łuczak, M., Łuczak, T., Cieścińska, C. & Czajkowski, R. (2013). General treatment of alopecia areata [Polish] *Przegl Dermatol.*, 100, 53–58.

Manolache, L., Petrescu-Seceleanu, D. & Benea, V. (2009). Alopecia areata and relationship with stressful events in children. *J Eur Acad Dermatol Venereol.*, 23, 107–109.

Mella, J. M., Perret, M. C., Manzotti, M., Catalano, H. N. & Guyatt, G. (2010). Efficacy and safety of finasteride therapy for androgenetic alopecia: a systematic review. *Arch Dermatol.*, 146, 1141–1150.

Messenger, A. G. & Rundegren, J. (2004). Minoxidil: mechanisms of action on hair growth. *Br J Dermatol.*, 150, 186–194.

Orecchia, G. & Rocchetti, G. A. (1995). Topical use of calcipotriol does not potentiate squaric acid dibutylester effectiveness in the treatment of alopecia areata. *J Dermatol Treat.*, 6, 21-23.

Paus, R. (2010). Exploring the "thyroid–skin connection": concepts, questions, and clinical relevance. *J Invest Dermatol.*, 130, 7–10.

Paus, R. (2011). A neuroendocrinological perspective on human hair follicle pigmentation. *Pigment Cell Melanoma Res.*, 24, 89–106.

Paus, R., Langan, E. A., Vidali, S., Ramot, Y. & Andersen, B. (2014). Neuroendocrinology of the hair follicle: principles and clinical perspectives. *Trends Mol Med.*, 20, 559–570.

Paus, R., Theoharides, T. C. & Arck, P. C. (2006). Neuroimmunoendocrine circuitry of the 'brain–skin connection'. *Trends Immunol.*, 27, 32–39.

Rajput, R. J. (2010). Controversy: Is there a role for adjuvants in the management of male pattern hair loss? *J Cutan Aesthet Surg.*, 3, 82-86.

Rogers, N. E. & Avram, M. R. (2008). Medical treatments for male and female pattern hair loss. *J Am Acad Dermatol*, 59, 547–566.

Saxena, K., Saxena, D. K. & Savant, S. S. (2016). Successful hair transplant outcome in cicatricial lichen planus of the scalp by combining scalp and beard hair along with platelet rich plasma. *J Cutan Aesthet Surg.*, *9*, 51–55.

Singh, S. (2015). Role of platelet-rich plasma in chronic alopecia areata: Our centre experience. *Indian J Plast Surg*, *48*, 57-59.

Slominski, A. T., Zmijewski, M. A., Skobowiat, C., Zbytek, B., Slominski, R. M. & Steketee, J. D. (2012). Sensing the environment: regulation of local and global homeostasis by the skin's neuroendocrine system. *Adv Anat Embryol Cell Biol.*, *212*, 1–115.

Spencer, D. K. (1998). The hormonal effects of diet on hair loss. In: Spencer DK editor. *The Bald Truth*. New York: Simon and Schuster Inc, p. 37-54.

Takahashi, T., Kamimura, A., Kagoura, M., Toyoda, M. & Morohashi, M. (2005). Investigation of the topical application of procyanidin oligomers from apples to identify their potential use as a hair-growing agent. *J Cosmet Dermatol.*, *4*, 245–249.

Takahashi, T., Kamimura, A., Yokoo, Y., Honda, S. & Watanabe, Y. (2001). The first clinical trial of topical application of procyanidin B-2 to investigate its potential as a hair growing agent. *Phytother Res.*, *15*, 331–336.

Tosti, A. (2007). Hair shaft disorders. in: tosti a, editor. Dermoscopy of hair and scalp: pathological and clinical correlation. Illustrated ed. usa: *CRC Press*, pp. 51-53.

Unger, W., Unger, R. & Wesley, C. (2008). The surgical treatment of cicatricial alopecia. *Dermatol Ther.*, *21*, 295–311.

Whiting, D. A. (1996). Chronic telogen effluvium: increased scalp hair shedding in middle-aged women. *J Am Acad Dermatol*. 35, 899–906.

Yong, A. A. & Unger, R. (2017). Resistance of Transplanted Hair Follicles to the Onslaught of Diffuse Alopecia Areata. *Am J Cosmet Surg.*, *34*, 70-72.

In: Alopecia
Editor: Pietro Gentile

ISBN: 978-1-53617-008-5
© 2020 Nova Science Publishers, Inc.

Chapter 5

GROWTH FACTOR RICH THERAPIES FOR THE TREATMENT OF HAIR LOSS

Megan A. Cole, PhD and John P. Cole[*], MD
Cole Hair Transplant Group, Alpharetta, GA, US

ABSTRACT

Traditional approaches to treating hair loss in men and women can be pharmacologic or surgical in nature. Prescription medications like finasteride have associated undesirable side effects including erectile dysfunction that may persist long after the treatment is discontinued, and some oral treatments are not recommended for use by female patients. Moreover, topical and oral drug-based treatments require long-term use for continuous effect. In this chapter, we will introduce four varieties of alternative treatments that have promising application in the hair regeneration field. Specifically, platelet rich plasma (PRP), amniotic-derived products, adipose-derived products, and exosomes are discussed in terms of their origin, isolation technique, and efficacy in treating hair loss. Of these treatment options, PRP and adipose-derived products have been evaluated most frequently in clinical applications, while amniotic-based products and exosomes have largely been screened at the cellular

---

[*] Corresponding Author's Email: forhair3@me.com.

level in a research capacity. All products have been associated with increased hair growth and induction of the telogen-to-anagen transition.

Keywords: platelet rich plasma, adipose mesenchymal stem cells, amniotic mesenchymal stem cells, exosomes

INTRODUCTION

Hair loss disorders like androgenetic alopecia and alopecia areata display relatively high rates of occurrence in both men and women. The extent of hair loss varies with etiology and, in some cases, with respect to age and gender. Likewise, the range of emotional burden on patients experiencing hair loss may extend from reduced self-esteem to mild anxiety or depression (Pemberton 2019). Moreover, hair loss may be a physical manifestation of an underlying systemic pathology, such as thyroid disease, systemic lupus erythematosus, or syphilis, or may occur secondary to a severe nutritional deficiency in protein, iron, zinc, or biotin. Consequently, therapies designed to stabilize remaining follicles or reverse the hair loss disorder entirely are highly desirable among health care professionals and consumers alike.

In order to determine what treatment(s) pose the greatest efficacy for patients suffering from hair loss, it is first critical to understand the hair growth cycle and the fundamental signaling pathways driving each stage. As shown in Figure 1, the hair cycle begins with a short period of apoptotic-driven hair follicle regression (catagen) that lasts approximately 2 weeks. During catagen, the deeper, highly proliferative structures of the hair follicle are lost, and the hair shaft and inner and outer root sheaths regress upwards. Following this period of regression, the hair follicle enters a state of relative quiescence (telogen) wherein the dermal papilla condenses, and the hair shaft is actively retained by a specialized junction complex located at the base of the bulge region. At this stage, the hair shaft is referred to as a "club" hair owing to the characteristic club-like morphology of its base. Late in telogen, the secondary hair germ is activated and proliferates rapidly, eventually elongating distally into the subcutaneous tissue where it surrounds the dermal papilla and establishes itself as a matrix of proliferative transit-amplifying cells. Cell differentiation programs are reactivated, a new inner root sheath and hair shaft are established, and melanogenesis ensues. Meanwhile, the club hair is shed (exogen) in an independently regulated process.

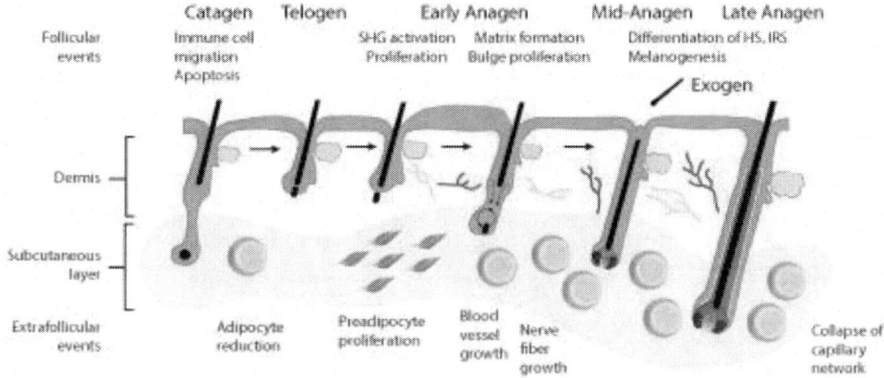

Figure 1. The hair growth cycle begins with upward regression of the outer root sheath and disappearance of highly proliferative cells in the deeper dermis. Mature adipocyte cell numbers decline, and composite skin thickness is reduced. In telogen, the hair follicle enters a state of relative quiescence wherein the shortened hair follicle is actively retained. Late in telogen, adipocyte precursors are induced to proliferate and commit to the adipocyte lineage. The intradermal adipocyte layer expands, the secondary hair germ is activated, and cells actively proliferate and migrate downwards into the subcutaneous tissue. By mid-anagen, a matrix of proliferative, transit amplifying cells encompass the dermal papilla, and in late anagen, a new inner and outer root sheath and hair shaft are established. Transition from anagen to catagen is marked by collapse of capillary network, lipolysis, and reduction in skin volume.

Many hair loss disorders (i.e., androgenetic alopecia, alopecia areata, and telogen effluvium) are characterized by concomitant increases and decreases in the durations of telogen and anagen, respectively. Therefore, signaling pathway(s) regulating the telogen to anagen transition are of particular importance in the context of hair loss reduction and/or reversal of such disorders. To date, two separate pathways, the canonical wingless (Wnt)/β-catenin cycle and the bone morphogenetic protein (BMP) pathway, have been linked to the hair follicle growth cycle. Competing gradients of their inhibitory and stimulatory signals fluctuate asynchronously, giving rise to an early "refractory" telogen follicle and a later "competent" telogen follicle primed to enter anagen (Geyfman et al. 2015).

The Wnt/β-catenin cycle effectively maintains bulge stem cells and secondary hair germ cells in their respective undifferentiated states via chronic inhibition of nuclear targets, specifically, members of the Tcf/Lef family of genes (Lowry et al. 2005). In dermal papilla, inhibition of these genes is regulated through the Frizzled (Fz) family of cell surface receptors, for which Wnt proteins are ligands. Binding of Wnt to Fz receptor complexes rescues β-catenin from proteasomal degradation, increasing cytoplasmic levels of β-catenin and facilitating its nuclear translocation where it associates with Lef1 DNA-binding proteins (Komiya and Habas 2008). The Wnt/β-catenin-directed transcriptional regulation of target genes is illustrated in Figure 2. Alternatively, regulation of Tcf3 in the bulge and secondary hair germ appears to function independent of the β-catenin interacting domain, sheltering cell populations within these regions from epidermal terminal differentiation cues to maintain their stem cell features (Merrill et al. 2001).

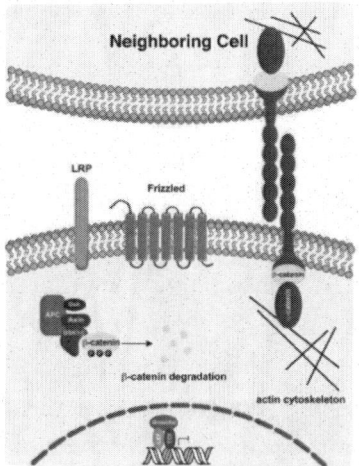 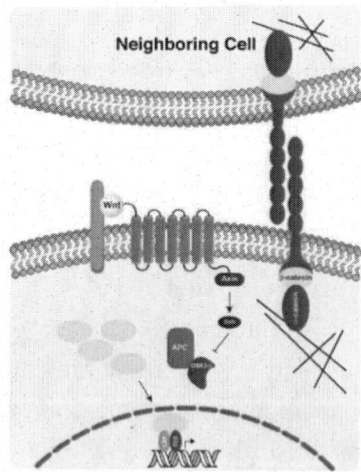

Figure 2. In the absence of Wnt, β-catentin is marked for degradation and nuclear targets Lef and Tcf are inhibited. When Wnt inhibition is released in late telogen, β-catentin, is 'rescued' and able to activate nuclear targets. *Shh* and its receptor *Ptc* are upregulated.

The BMP pathway regulates crosstalk between the endothelial and mesenchymal cellular compartments; BMP expressed by fibroblasts and keratinocytes during early (refractory) telogen inhibits Wnt expression through association with the BMP receptor (BMPR-1A) that is selectively expressed in the secondary hair germ (Botchkarev et al. 2001). Transition from refractory to competent telogen is similarly directed by interdepartmental BMP signaling. Late in telogen, the hair follicle epithelium and dermal papilla express noggin, which competitively inhibits BMP to actively reduce its association with BMPR-1A. Consequently, local inhibition of Wnt is released, and downstream effectors of the Wnt/β-catenin pathway are activated, leading to one of the earliest hallmarks of hair follicle formation, upregulation of sonic hedgehog (Shh) and its receptor Patched (Ptc) (Lo Celso et al. 2004). Additionally, in late (competent) telogen, dermal papilla cells begin producing fibroblast growth factor 7/10 (Fgf7/10) ligands that stimulate the secondary hair germ and, to a much lesser extent, the bulge to proliferate via FGFR2-11 1b binding events. In contrast, the secretory profile of dermal papilla in early (refractory) telogen is dominated by FGF18 expression that actively inhibits bulge cells through its association with FGFR3.

Existing pharmacological interventions designed to reduce hair loss and/or improve hair growth target one or both of the pathways presented above. Oral finasteride formulations, for example, are considered Wnt upregulators and have been associated with increased scalp hair density in men diagnosed with androgenetic alopecia. As a selective 5α-reductase, finasteride inhibits the conversion of testosterone (T) into the more potent dihydrotestosterone (DHT) that binds androgen receptors with a greater affinity. Androgen receptors (AR) are overexpressed in the dermal papilla of patients suffering from androgenetic alopecia, and in their T- or DHT-bound state function as ligand-dependent transcription factors that interact with β-catenin to inhibit Wnt-mediated transcriptional activity (Kitagawa et al. 2009). Since finasteride reduces the relative concentration of DHT, nuclear translocation events of the AR-DHT complex are reduced and Wnt signaling events are improved.

Like other prescription hair loss medications, finasteride requires consistent, ongoing use for lasting results, but the number of undesirable side effects often restrict long term patient compliance. Therefore, alternative treatments of natural origins have become a standard of care in the hair loss industry. Products such as platelet rich plasma, amniotic- and adipose-derived products, and exosomes deliver high quantities of growth factors and cytokines to stimulate hair growth via the Wnt/β-catenin and BMP pathways. In this chapter, we will provide an overview of each of these products to discuss how they are sourced, prepared, and delivered; explain their connection to the hair growth pathway(s); evaluate their established efficacy at present and address their relevant safety concerns.

Platelet Rich Plasma

Platelet rich plasma (PRP) represents an autologous source of growth factors, chemokines and cytokines, antimicrobial proteins, membrane glycoproteins, clotting factors and their inhibitors, and fibrinolytic factors and their inhibitors that have been applied to effect positive outcomes in an abundance of disease states (Nurden 2011). Indeed, PRP has proven beneficial in speeding wound healing (Chicharro-Alcántara et al. 2018), modulating inflammatory skin conditions such as atopic dermatitis and psoriasis (Cho et al. 2014, Chakravdhanula et al. 2016), and the improving standard of care in autoimmune disorders including ulcerative colitis and rheumatoid arthritis (da Silva et al. 2017, Tong et al. 2017). The propensity for incorporating PRP in clinical trials across such a broad spectrum of health care needs likely stems from the simplicity of the collection procedure and the minimal risk associated with the use of an autologous blood-based product.

During PRP production, whole blood is collected from the patient and subjected to differential centrifugation to sediment cellular constituents on the basis of specific gravity. Standardization of the PRP collection protocol from one clinic to the next, however, dissolves rapidly beyond the venous blood draw. For example, PRP can be prepared using either the PRP method or the buffy-coat method, which differ in the sequence of the 'high' and 'low' speed centrifugation steps, the duration of each spin, and the temperature at which the steps are completed, leading to discrepancies in the degree of platelet concentration above baseline (Dhurat and Sukesh 2014). Several commercial kits are now available to regulate the foldchange in platelet concentration; however, the upper limit is inevitably bounded by the absolute quantity of platelets in the whole blood sample provided by the individual patient, meaning that variations in product quality from one patient to the next are unavoidable. Furthermore, the extent to which commercial devices concentrate platelets range from 2.5× to 9× above baseline. The operator is advised to conduct a personalized product review and base the purchase on desired clinical needs.

In clinical applications, autologous PRP can either be used directly in its native state (A-PRP) or activated with calcium or thrombin to release the growth factor-rich contents of its alpha granules prior to delivery (AA-PRP). With respect to hair growth, both modalities have proven beneficial; scalp injections with A-PRP have produced increases in hair density ranging from 13% to 31% over baseline values 3 months after treatment (Takikawa et al. 2011, Gentile et al. 2017). Likewise, improvements in hair density have ranged from 18% to 29% above baseline at approximately 3 months to as much as 56% above baseline at 6 months following AA-PRP scalp injections (Gentile et al. 2015, Cervelli et al. 2014, Gkini et al. 2014). Notably, the degree of hair density improvement was dependent on the commercial system used to prepare the PRP (Gentile et al. 2017). Improvements in hair growth have been observed in both male and female subjects, with the latter maintaining satisfaction in the treatment results at 6-month return consultations, where, on average, a twofold increase in hair density was recorded (Tawfik and Osman 2017).

Microscopic evaluation of scalp harvested from patients receiving AA-PRP injections have demonstrated increased epidermal thickness and perifollicular vascularization in addition to the increased number of hair follicles discussed above (Cervelli et al. 2014). Such modifications in scalp histology may be attributable to the specific growth factors and cytokines present in platelets and made immediately available for cellular uptake following activation with calcium or thrombin or lysed via sonication (Cole et al. 2017). Specifically, insulin-like growth factor 1 (IGF-1) has been shown to affect follicular proliferation, tissue remodeling, the hair regrowth cycle, and follicular differentiation (Weger and Schlake 2005), while isoforms of platelet-derived growth factor (PDGF) are known to induce entry into the anagen phase leading to upregulation of signaling molecules related to hair follicle differentiation including Shh, Lef-1, and Wnt5a (Tomita et al. 2006). Epidermal growth factor (EGF) stimulates the proliferation of basal keratinocytes and outer root sheath cells but has an inhibitory effect on cells in the hair bulb (Mark and Chan 2003). Meanwhile, vascular endothelial growth factor (VEGF) induces perifollicular angiogenesis, and basic fibroblast growth factor (bFGF or FGF-2) promotes hair growth by inducing the telogen-to-anagen transition (Lin et al. 2015). For a complete list of growth factors, mitogenic agents, and additional components found in platelet alpha granules, the reader may refer to the 2011 *Thrombosis and Haemostasis* article on the subject (Nurden 2011).

Primary dermal papilla cell lines extracted from human scalp tissue have shown increased proliferation, increased Bcl-2 and FGF-7 levels, activated ERK and Akt proteins, and upregulation of β-catenin when cultured in an AA-PRP supplemented growth medium (Li et al. 2012). Controlled expression of these proteins and pathways have significant implications in hair regeneration since, as established in the introduction section of this chapter, each correlates with a positive impact on hair growth, including cellular proliferation to prolong the anagen phase (FGF-7) (Greco et al. 2009), inducing cell growth (ERK activation) (Robinson and Cobb 1997), hair follicle development (β-catenin) (Lichtenberger et al. 2016), and suppression of apoptotic cues (Bcl-2 release and Akt activation) (Ahmad et al. 1999, Yang et al. 2016).

Although standardization of individual growth factor concentrations within autologous PRP is inherently unachievable, and the optimized ratios of these growth factors is yet to be known, clinical application of the product is generally agreed to be beneficial a pose no risk beyond those associated with receiving an injection. Moreover, decellularized versions of platelet lysate with regulated batch-to-batch similarity are already available for both clinical and research purposes.

Amniotic Products

Amniotic products encompass those derived from the innermost layer of the human placenta (i.e., the amnion) or from the amniotic fluid of healthy, full-term pregnancies. Ethical considerations, such as those encountered in embryonic stem cell therapies, are circumvented given that retrieval of the products requires maternal consent of material that would otherwise be discarded and poses no additional risk to the live birth. Amniotic products may be used in either a cellular or acellular format depending on the source material and method of preparation. Cellular versions, for example, are routinely prepared via mechanical removal of the amnion from the placenta by blunt dissection under aseptic techniques (Niknejad et al., 2011). Screening of the tissue for blood-borne pathogens, including hepatitis B and hepatitis C, syphilis, and human immunodeficiency virus (HIV) followed by lyophilization or cryopreservation yields allogenic tissue grafts for direct use in patients. Alternatively, acellular products may be prepared from conditioned media using amniotic fluid- or membrane-derived mesenchymal stem cells. The media is "conditioned" by first expanding the cell population to 60-70% confluency under standard cell culture conditions then replacing the serum-supplemented culture media with serum-free media to be enriched with growth factors, cytokines, and immunomodulatory factors by the cells until they reach 100% confluency (Dowling and Clynes 2010). Additionally, one study has shown that amniotic fluid preparations from at least three commercial vendors (PalinGen, FloGraft, and Genesis) contain varying levels of growth factors and hyaluronan but no evidence of mesenchymal stem cells (Panero et al. 2019).

Cryopreservation of amniotic membrane sectioned as large as 10 cm × 10 cm has been shown to contain viable cell populations in both the stromal and epithelial layers (Perepelkin et al. 2015), making these allogenic tissue grafts a particularly attractive resource in the field of regenerative medicine given their extremely low immunogenicity profiles and high secretion of growth factors and cytokines that affect cellular growth and proliferation. Indeed, the multipotent amniotic epithelial and mesenchymal stromal cells possess embryonic ectoderm and mesoderm cell lineages, respectively, and, like other placental organs, are deemed "immunoprivileged" (Akle et al. 1981). They express low levels of major histocompatibility complex (MHC) class I surface antigens and no MHC class II surface antigens (Niknejad et al. 2008). Consequently, dehydrated amniotic membrane allografts have proven to be a safe, efficacious adjunct to dural closures for craniotomies and transsphenoidal surgeries (Eichberg et al. 2018) as well as a stand-alone therapy for improved lower extremity wound closure in diabetic patients when applied in a concentrated, granularized form (Bazrafshan et al. 2014, Werber and Martin 2013).

The therapeutic benefits derived from amniotic products may be attributed to their contents and structure; cellular formats are delivered with both the multipotent stem cells and a scaffold in which they can grow, migrate, and adhere. Amniotic membrane consists of fibroblasts, growth factors, collagens III, IV, V, and VII, fibronectin, and laminin. Together these factors modulate growth factor and cytokine levels, suppress pain, fibrosis, and bacterial growth, and promote wound healing (Toda et al. 2007). Likewise, amniotic fluid contains a vast assortment of nutrients (i.e., carbohydrates, proteins and peptides, lipids, electrolytes, and hormones), growth factors (i.e., TGF-α, TGF-β1, and FGF), antimicrobial peptides, and hyaluronic acid (Underwood et al. 2005).

Cell lines treated with amniotic products overwhelmingly respond in a positive manner. Keratinocytes cultured with human amniotic epithelial stem cell- (HAESC) conditioned media or co-cultured in the presence of HAESCs exhibit accelerated migration and proliferation secondary to upregulation of proteins controlled along the ERK, JNK, Akt signaling pathway (Zhao et al. 2016). Furthermore, hyaluronic acid has proven important for re-epithelialization, and the high content within amniotic fluid accelerates the process in wound healing (Nyman et al. 2013). Additionally, treatment of tenocytes with amniotic suspension allografts or conditioned media thereof increases cell density, leads to robust migration and matrix deposition, and alters inflammatory targets (Kimmerling et al. 2018). Finally, amniotic fluid-derived mesenchymal stem cell conditioned media has been shown to enhance dermal fibroblast proliferation and accelerate wound healing leading to faster hair regeneration and growth (Yoon et al. 2010). The shift may be attributable to elevated FGF-7 levels in the dermis following treatment (Seo et al. 2016).

The use of amniotic stem cell-conditioned media has particular relevance for regenerative hair treatments. As mentioned previously, conditioned medias eliminate the potential concerns associated with cell-based therapies, albeit such risks are already minimal given the immunopriviledged status of amniotic cell lines. Conditioned media can be evaluated for dosage, efficacy, and side effects in a process identical to existing pharmaceuticals. Moreover, they can be mass produced in an economical and targeted manner; mesenchymal stem cells can be manipulated to overexpress compounds with greater clinical significance. For example, overexpression of NANOG in amniotic fluid mesenchymal stem cells has been shown to increase the positive regulators of hair follicle regrowth twofold (Park et al. 2019). NANOG is the transcription regulator responsible for preserving embryonic cell "stemness" (i.e., high rates of self-renewal without concomitant differentiation) (Hyslop et al. 2005). As shown by Park et al., overexpression of NANOG in amniotic fluid mesenchymal stem cells produces a conditioned media that accelerates the telogen-to-anagen transition in hair follicles and increases hair follicle density to a rate comparable to treatment with 2% minoxidil.

Adipose Mesenchymal Stem Cell Products

Adipose-based treatments may be considered a hybrid of amniotic products and PRP treatments in that they may either contain a stem cell population or merely the conditioned media thereof, as in amniotic-based products, and cellular versions are derived from the patient's own tissue (i.e., adipose treatments, like PRP treatments, are autologous). Since the cell population is autologous, reinjection into the source patient poses no inherent risk of tissue rejection or infection so long as sterile conditions are maintained throughout the entire processing procedure, which is outlined below.

Production of an adipose-based therapy begins with lipoaspiration. At this juncture, the collected adipose tissue can be processed by a commercially available device such as PureGraft or Kerastem Celulation, both of which are manufactured by the Bimini group and are approved for purchase in Europe and Japan; Kerastem has not yet received FDA clearance in the United States but has successfully completed a phase II clinical study. Alternatively, the lipoaspirate may be washed with normal saline and processed via mechanical or enzymatic techniques to establish an autologous population of adipose-derived stromal vascular cells (ADSVC) that should be sorted according to cell surface markers such that a reproducible and consistent composition of cells are attained (Li et al. 2013). Immediate reinjection of this cell population into the source patient qualifies as minimal tissue processing so long as the cell population is not expanded in culture, in which case the treatment would be considered an advanced therapy medical product and fall under restrictions set forth by the European Medicine Agency (Gentile 2019).

ADSVC encompass multiple cell types, including adipose-derived stem cells (ADSC), mesenchymal and endothelial progenitor cells, leukocyte subtypes, lymphatic cells, pericytes, and vascular smooth muscle cells. They hold unrivaled potential as a therapeutic source in regenerative medicine owing to the relative abundance and facile removal of adipose tissue from patients and the simplistic nature of isolating higher quantities of stem cells from adipose tissue relative to bone marrow. Moreover, ADSC support superior improvement in inflammation, granulation tissue re-organization, and collagen deposition in full thickness wounds relative to bone marrow-derived stem cell treatments (Aboulhoda and Abd El Fattah 2018). The outperformance of ADSC-based therapies may be attributable to their extensive proliferative capacities, high recovery yields, and enhanced capability to exist (Fraser et al. 2006, Peng et al. 2008, Zhu et al. 2012). Indeed, ADSC can withstand cryopreservation for at least 6 months (Marques-Curtis et al. 2015). The cells retain their potential to differentiate into mesenchymal lineage cells and to secrete a variety of cytokines and growth factors, including hepatocyte growth factor (HGF), VEGF, PDGF, and IGF (Kinniard et al. 2004, L PK 2019).

ADSC and descendants thereof are particularly relevant to the field of hair regeneration given that adipose lineage cells contribute differentially to the hair follicle growth cycle. ADSC, for example, have a stimulatory effect on dermal papilla cells to promote hair follicle cycling (Won et al. 2010, Plikus et al. 2008). Defective generation of precursor adipocytes precludes hair follicle stem cell activation to such an extent that the mere presences of immature adipocytes is now considered necessary and sufficient to induce the telogen-to-anagen transition (Festa et al. 2011). Mature adipocytes, on the other hand, inhibit hair follicle progression (Schmidt and Horsley 2012, Tang and Lane 2012, Shook et al. 2016). These seemingly antagonistic, population-dependent effects on follicles are well synchronized with the stages of the hair cycle. As depicted in Figure 1, multiple changes within the skin occur during the hair follicle regenerative cycle (Blanpain and Fuchs 2006). Early in anagen, the intradermal adipocyte layer expands, effectively doubling the overall skin thickness (Butcher 1934), and by mid-anagen 20-40% of the increased mature adipocyte population is comprised of newly-differentiated adipocyte progenitor cells (Rivera-Gonzalez 2016, Zhang et al. 2016). Local levels of adipocyte-derived BMP2 similarly rise during anagen and exerts an inhibitory effect on hair follicle stem cells during telogen to suppress hair growth (Guerrero-Juarez and Plikus 2018, Plikus et al. 2008). Conversely, periodic expression of BMP4 in the intra-follicular epithelium, secondary hair germ, dermal papilla and adjacent extra-follicular dermal fibroblasts promotes adipocyte lineage commitment in ADSCs and is induced in the cells during their differentiation (Gustafson et al. 2013, Plikus et al. 2008).

The beneficial effect of ADVSCs and conditioned media of these cell populations as an alternative treatment in the hair regeneration field is well established (Epstein and Epstein 2018). Improvements in hair regeneration evidenced by increased hair density and diameter have been noted in male and female subjects following ADVSC scalp injections (Anderi et al. 2018). Likewise, significant increases in hair count have been observed without concurrent changes in the fraction of hair follicles in the anagen or telogen stage of growth when 1.0 mL cm^{-2} mixtures of purified adipose tissue (PureGraft), ADSCs (Kerastem Celulation), and Ringer's lactate solution were injected into patient scalps (Perez-Meza et al. 2017). Additional studies have indicated that combined ADSC/adipose therapies improve graft quality with notable increases in capillary density, enhancements of angiogenesis and adipocyte differentiation, and suppression of apoptotic pathways via VEGF-A and IGF-1 expression (Zhu et al. 2010). Indeed, combination style therapies appear to extend beyond hair regenerative therapies; application of a keratin scaffold in conjunction with human adipose stem cells shortens wound healing time, accelerates epithelialization, and promotes wound remodeling relative to adipose stem cells delivered in solution (Lin et al. 2018).

Therapies derived from ADVSC conditioned media have afforded similar improvements in hair regeneration. For example, ADSC conditioned media (ADSC-CM) has been shown to significantly enhance the proliferation of human dermal papilla cells through activation of ERK and Akt signaling pathways (Won et al. 2019). Two additional studies have examined the efficacy of a commercially available ADSC-CM (NGAL, Prostemics Research Institute, South Korea). One found a significant increase in hair density and thickness in female patients who received a 3-month course of weekly NGAL injections (Shin et al. 2015), while the second noted significant increases in hair count following 4 – 6 NGAL injection sessions spaced (Fukuoka et al. 2017).

As with conditioned media from amniotic stem cells, research has shown that the secretome in ADSC-CM can be optimized for a given therapeutic application (Sagaradze et al. 2019). In particular, pre-conditioning ADSC with vitamin C, PDGF, UV-B exposure, or hypoxic culture conditions enhanced the hair regenerative ability of conditioned media by accelerating anagen induction (Jin and Sung 2016). Likewise, pre-conditioning of ADSC with minoxidil or udenafil, a phosphodiesterase type 5 (PEE$_5$) inhibitor produces conditioned media that, upon injection, accelerates the telogen-to-anagen transition (Choi et al. 2018, Choi and Sung 2019).

Exosomes

Exosomes are emerging as an alternative, cell-free therapeutic in regenerative medicine that pose minimal risk to patients. These small (50 – 150 nm), membrane-bound particles are a subtype of extracellular vesicles (EV) and, like other EVs (i.e., microvesicles and apoptotic bodies), are recognized for their physiological and pathological relevance in cell-cell signaling (Mitelbrunn and Sánchez-Madrid 2012). Specifically, exosomes have the ability to influence a number of signaling pathways that modulate cellular processes, including proliferation, differentiation, migration, or even programed cell death (Colombo et al. 2014, Jiang et al. 2017).

Exosomes originate via the endocytic pathway. Inward budding of the plasma membrane or fusion of vesicles gives rise to early endosomes that may subsequently undergo a second inward budding to produce multiple smaller vesicles within the original vesicle. Terminology associated with this process is as follows; the host vesicle is referred to as a multivesicular endosome (MVE), and its cargo are known as intraluminal vesicles (ILVs). ILV generated in this process may either be marked for lysosomal degradation or secreted into the extracellular space by exocytosis, where the vesicles are renamed 'exosomes' and function as carriers of proteins, lipids, and genetic material to distant tissues (Jeppesen et al. 2019, Tkack and Théry 2016).

Interestingly, the intracellular machinery involved in exosome production is cell-specific. Different families of molecules have been identified in modulating the formation and secretion of ILVs and contribute to the existence of exosome sub-types (Kowal et al. 2014). Specifically, exosome secretion is predominantly regulated by Rab GTPase in a pathway involving Endosomal Sorting Complexes Required for Transport (ESCRT), although the process can occur in an ESCRT-independent manner (Vallarroya-Beltri et al. 2014, Van Niel et al. 2018).

Regardless of the specific pathway, lipids and members of the tetraspanin family are heavily involved, and the presence of tetraspanins CD63, CD81, CD9 serve as classical exosome-specific surface markers (Théry et al. 2002, Tkach et al. 2017)

Multiple cellular materials may be considered sources of exosomes (i.e., biological fluids or conditioned cell culture media). However, isolation and purification of a single exosome population from the wealth of EVs present in these products can be time and labor intensive (Gardiner et al. 2016). Ultracentrifugation followed by sucrose density gradient ultracentrifugation remains a gold standard in isolating a relatively homogeneous size population of exosomes (György et al. 2011). Although the first ultracentrifugation process may be completed in a matter of hours, the sucrose density gradient separation requires an overnight ultracentrifugation ($\geq$ 14 hr); exosomes have been proven to float at densities of 1.15 to 1.19 g mL^{-1} on a continuous sucrose gradient facilitating their separation from vesicles of endoplasmic reticulum- or Golgi body-origin that float at densities of 1.18 to 1.25 g mL^{-1} and 1.05 to 1.12 g mL^{-1}, respectively (Théry et al. 2006).

Given the extensive timeframe required for exosome isolation by ultracentrifugation protocol and the growing clinical demand for reliable exosome recovery techniques, several commercial options have emerged. Many of these products utilize sedimentation to separate exosomes from non-target factors within the sample but have proven subpar to conventional ultracentrifugation or immunoaffinity methods with respect to the number of exosome particles recovered relative to total protein measured (Brett et al. 2017). In essence, the sedementation-based kits experience high degrees on non-specific protein absorption along with exosome collection. However, a commercial kit based on size exclusion chromatography separation methods proves comparable to ultracentrifugation techniques so long as collected exosome fractions are subsequently pooled and concentrated (Lobb et al. 2015).

Potential clinical applications for exosomes are abundant. Exosomes collected from the conditioned media of bone marrow mesenchymal stem cells (MSCs) have been shown to suppress inflammation and inhibit mitochondrial-induced apoptosis in chondrocytes via the p38, ERK, Akt signaling pathway (Qi et al. 2019). Consequently, exosomes derived from bone marrow MSCs have recognized therapeutic potential in osteoarthritis and other degenerative diseases (Chang et al. 2018). Moreover, exosomes from bone marrow MSCs have proven to alleviate liver fibrosis effectively in rats; exosome treatment reduced collagen accumulation, enhanced liver function, and increased hepatocyte regeneration (Rong et al. 2019). Exosomes from culture supernatant of other cell populations have similarly demonstrated positive therapeutic results. With respect to skin wound healing, exosomes derived from adipose MSCs, human amniotic epithelial cells, and human umbilical cord MSCs have led to improved fibroblast function, enhanced fibroblast proliferation and migration, and activation of intracellular fibroblast β-catenin and Wnt4 pathways, respectively (Liu et al. 2018).

Understanding the role of exosomes in hair growth rejuvenation is gaining momentum and is summarized nicely in a recent review by Carrasco (Carraco et al. 2019). Exosomes harvested from conditioned media of dermal papilla (DP) cells and bone marrow MSCs have been associated with positive effects on hair growth, cycling, and regeneration. Namely, treatment of mice with DP-derived exosomes induced a telogen-to-anagen transition and prolonged anagen (Kwack et al. 2019). DP exosome injections have also been linked with elevated β-catenin and Shh levels in mouse tissue as well as increased outer root sheath cell proliferation and migration (Zhou et al. 2018). Additionally, miRNA within DP-exosomes can regulate hair follicle stem cell (HFSC) proliferation by targeting *LEF1*, a key transcription factor in inducing HFSC differentiation and promoting β-catenin translocation (Yan et al. 2019). Lastly, exosomes from bone marrow MSC also have proven have the potential to activate DP cells, prolong cell survival, induce GF activation, and promote hair growth (Rajendran et al. 2017). Indeed, exosomes have demonstrated definitive therapeutic potential and should be the focus of much future research.

CONCLUSION

A diverse selection of alternative therapies is rapidly gaining traction in the field of regenerative medicine. Some of these products have already infiltrated the hair loss treatment market and are demonstrating promising results. Numerous small-scale clinical trials have been conducted using autologous PRP, activated autologous PRP, adipose mesenchymal stem cells with or without autologous adipose tissue grafts, or conditioned media from cultured adipose mesenchymal stem cells or amniotic mesenchymal stem cells. No serious side effects have been noted in the studies reviewed herein. However, methods to standardize the active ingredients within these therapies are lacking at present. Therefore, side by side comparisons of results attained in different clinics are limited. In particular, the baseline and final concentration of platelets in PRP varies not only from one patient to the next but within a single donor depending on the commercial device used to prepare the injectable product. Moreover, no single 'activation' protocol exists for isolating growth factor-rich contents from the alpha granules of platelets in therapies wherein autologous activated PRP is applied. Nevertheless, the consensus among original research papers and review articles alike is that PRP in either form has a positive impact on hair growth, thought the extent to which that claim is true has yet to reach an agreed upon level.

Clinical studies using amniotic- or adipose-derived therapies similarly lack a standardized method of preparation. Treatments composed of either such product, however, have the added dilemma of which component(s) to include: cells, matrix, conditioned media, or some combination thereof. Additionally, in preparing conditioned media, factors such as hypoxic culture conditions, irradiation with ultraviolet light, or exogenous supplements can be used to modify protein composition. Therefore, more work is needed to identify how these treatment lines can be formatted for optimized hair regeneration in clinical practice.

Exosome therapies have the highest economic burden but may have superior clinical performance. Isolation of these potent extracellular vesicles is complex; they must be sorted from an abundance of membranous structures from cell culture media and confirmed as target product visually and on the basis of surface proteins. Consequently, the variety of isolation protocols are numerous, as are the cell lines from which exosomes may be attained. However, exosomes that have been isolated from bone marrow mesenchymal cell media and dermal papilla cell media significantly improve proliferation of dermal papilla, outer root sheath, and hair follicle stem cells. Therefore, a standardized clinical trial wherein the efficacy of exosomes as a therapeutic tool for treating hair loss disorders would prove highly valuable to clinicians and the scientific community at large.

REFERENCES

Aboulhoda, Basma Emad, Adb El Fattah, Shereen. 2018. "Bone marrow-derived versus adipose-derived stem cells in wound healing: value and route of administration." *Cell and Tissue Research* 374:285-302.

Ahmad, Shakeel, Singh, Nadia, Glazer, Robert I. 1999. "Role of AKT1 in 17β-estradiol- and insulin-like growth factor I (IGF-I)-dependent proliferation and prevention of apoptosis in MCF-7 breast carcinoma cells." *Molecular and Cellular Pharmacology* 58:425-30.

Anderi, Rami, Makdissy, Nehman, Azar, Albert, Hamade, Aline. 2018. "Cellular therapy with human autologous adipose-derived adult cells of stromal vascular fraction for alopecia areata." *Stem Cell Research & Therapy* 9:141.

Akle, C. A., Adinolfi, M., Welsh K. I., Leibowitz, S., McColl, I. 1981. "Immunogenicity of human amniotic epithelial cells after transplantation into volunteers." *Lancet* 2:1003-5.

Bazrafshan, Ameneh, Owji, Mohammad, Yazdani, Maryam, Varedi, Masoumeh. 2014. "Activation of mitosis and angiogenesis in diabetes-impaired wound healing by processed human amniotic fluid." *Journal of Surgical Research* 188:545-52.

Blanpain, Cédric and Fuchs, Elaine. 2006. "Epidermal stem cells of the skin." *Annual Review of Cell and Developmental Biology* 22:339-73.

Botchkarev, Vladimir A., Botchkareva, Natalia V., Nakamura, Motonobu, Huber, Otmar, Funa, Keiko, Lauster, Roland, Paus, Ralf, Gilchrest, Barbara A. 2001. "Noggin is required for induction of the hair follicle growth phase in postnatal skin." *FASEB Journal* 15:2205-14.

Brett, Sabine I., Lucien, Fabrice, Guo, Charles, Williams, Karla C., Kim, Yohan, Durfee, Paul N., Brinker, C. J., Chin, Joseph I., Yang, Jun, Leong, Hon S. 2017. "Immunoaffinitiy based methods are superior to kits for purification of prostate derived extracellular vesicles from plasma samples." *The Prostate* 77:1335-43.

Butcher, Earl O. 1934. "The hair cycles in the albino rat." *The Anatomical Record* 61:5-19.

Carrasco, Elisa, Soto-Heredero, Gonzalo, Mittelbrunn, María. 2019. "The role of extracellular vesicles in cutaneous remodeling and hair follicle dynamics." *International Journal of Molecular Sciences* 20:2758.

Cervelli, Valerio, Garcovich, Simone, Bielli, Alessandra, Cervelli, G., Curcio, B. C., Scioli, Maria Giovanna, Orlandi, Augusto, Gentile, Pietro. 2014. "The effect of autologous activated platelet rich plasma (AA-PRP) injection on pattern hair loss: Clinical and histomorphometric evaluation." *BioMed Research International* 760709:9.

Chakravdhanula, Uma, Anbarasu, Kavitha, Verma, Vinod Kumar, Beevi, Syed Sultan. 2016. "Clinical efficacy of platelet rich plasma in combination with methotrexate in chronic plaque psoriatic patients." *Dermatologic Therapy* 29:446-50.

Chang, Yu-Hsun, Wu, Kung-Chi, Harn, Horng-Jyh, Lin, Shinn-Zong, Ding, Dah-Ching. 2018. "Exosomes and stem cells in degenerative disease diagnosis and therapy." *Cell Transplantation* 27:349-63.

Chicharro-Alcántara, Deborah, Rubio-Zaragoza, Mónica, Damiá-Giménez, Elena, Carrillo-Poveda, José, Cuervo-Serrato, Belén, Peláez-Gorrea, Pau, Sopena-Juncosa, Joaquín J. 2018. "Platelet rich plasma: New insights for cutaneous wound healing management." *Journal of Functional Biomaterials* 9:10.

Cho, S. M., Kim, M. E., Kim, J. Y., Park, J. C., Nahm, D. H., 2014. "Clinical efficacy of autologous plasma therapy for atopic dermatis." *Dermatology* 228:71-77.

Choi, Nahyun, Shin, Soyoung, Song, Sun U., Sung, Jong-Hyuk. 2018. "Minoxidil promotes hair growth through stimulation of growth factor release from adipose-derived stem cells." *International Journal of Molecular Sciences* 19:691.

Choi, Nahyun, Sung, Jong-Hyuk. 2019. "Udenafil inducs the hair growth effect of adipose-derived stem cells." *Biomolecules & Therapeutics* 27:404-13.

Cole, John P., Cole, Megan A., Insalaco, Chiara, Cervelli, Valerio, Gentile, Pietro. 2017. "Alopecia and platelet-derived therapies." *Stem Cell Investigation* 4:88.

Da Silva, Francesca A. R., Rodrigues, Bruno Lima, Huber, Stephany Cares, Júnior, Jose L. R. C., Lana, Jose F. S. D., de Lima Montalvão, Silmara Aparecida, Luzo, Ângela C. M., Ayrizono, Maria L. S., Coy, Cláudio, S. R., Leal, Raquel Franco, Annichino-Bizzacchi, Joyce Maria. 2017. "The use of platelet rich plasma in the treatment of refractory Crohn's disease." *International Journal of Clinical and Experimental Medicine* 10:7533-42.

Dhurat, Rachita and Sukesh, M. S. 2014. "Principles and methods of preparation of platelet-rich plasma: A review and author's perspective." *Journal of Cutaneous and Aesthetic Surgery* 7:189-97.

Dowling, Paul, Clynes, Martin. 2010. "Conditioned media from cell lines: A complementary model to clinical specimens for the discovery of disease-specific biomarkers." *Proteomics* 11:794-804.

Eichberg, Daniel G., Ali, Sheikh C., Buttrick, Simon S., Komotar, Ricardo J. 2018. "The use of dehydrated amniotic membrane allograft for augmentation of dural closure in craniotomies and endoscopic endonasal transsphenoidal surgeries." *British Journal of Neurosurgery* 32:516-20.

Epstein, Gorana Kuka, Epstein, Jeffrey S. 2018. "Mesenchymal stem cells and stromal vascular fraction for hair loss." *Facial Plastic Surgery Clinics of North America* 26:503-11.

Festa, Eric, Fretz, Jackie, Berry, Ryan, Schmidt, Barbara, Rodeheffer, Matthew, Horowitz, Mark, Horsley, Valerie. 2011. "Adipocyte lineage cells contribute to the skin stem cell niche to drive hair cycling." *Cell* 146:761-71.

Fraser, John K., Wulur, Isabella, Alfonso, Zeni, Hedrick, Marc H. 2006. "Fat tissue: an underappreciated source of stem cells for biotechnology." *Trends in Biotechnology* 24:150-54.

Fukuoka, Hirotaro, Narita, Keigo, Suga, Hirotaka. 2017. "Hair regeneration therapy: Application of adipose-derived stem cells." *Current Stem Cell Research & Therapy* 12:531-34.

Gardiner, Chris, Di Vizio, Dolores, Sahoo, Susmita, Thery, Clotilde, Witwer, Kenneth W., Wauben Marca, Hill, Andrew F. 2016. "Techniques used for the isolation and characterization of extracellular vesicles: results of a worldwide survey." *Journal of Extracellular Vesicles* 5:32945.

Gentile, Pietro. 2019. "Human adipose tissue derived follicle stem cells in adrogenic alopecia." *International Journal of Molecular Sciences* 20:3446.

Gentile, Pietro, Cole, John P., Cole, Megan A., Garcovich, Simone, Bielli, Alessandra, Scioli, Maria Giovanna, Orlandi, Augusto, Insalaco, Chiara, Cervelli, Valerio. 2017. "Evaluation of not-activated and activated PRP in hair loss treatment: Role of growth factor and cytokine concentrations obtained by different collection systems." *International Journal of Molecular Sciences* 18:408.

Gentile, Pietro, Garcovich, Simone. 2019. "Androgenic alopecia and hair loss: Wnt pathway, growth-factor, and mesenchymal stem cell signaling impact analysis on cell growth and hair follicle development." *Cell* 8:466.

Gentile, Pietro, Garcovich, Simone, Bielli, Alessandra, Scioli, Maria Giovannna, Orlandi, Augusto, Cervelli, Valerio. 2015. "The effect of platelet-rich plasma in hair regrowth: A randomized placebo-controlled trial" *Stem Cells Translational Medicine* 4:1317-23.

Geyfman, Mikhail, Plikus, Maksim V., Treffeisen, Elsa, Andersen, Bogi, Paus, Ralf. 2015. "Resting no more: re-defining telogen, the maintenance stage of the hair growth cycle." *Biological Reviews* 90:1179-96.

Gkini, Maria-Angeliki, Kouskoukis, Alexandros-Efstratios, Tripsianis, Gregory, Rigopoulos, Dimitris, Kouskoukis, Konstantinos. 2014. "Study of platelet-rich plasma injections in the treatment of androgenetic alopecia through a one-year period." *Journal of Cutaneous and Aesthetic Surgery* 7:213-19.

Greco, Valentina, Chen, Ting, Rendl, Michael, Schober, Markus, Pasolli, H. Amalia, Stokes, Nicole, dela Cruz-Racelis, June, Fuchs, Elaine. 2008. "A two-step mechanism for stem cell activation during hair regeneration." *Cell Stem Cell* 4:155-69.

Guerrero-Juarez, Christian F. and Plikus, Maksim V. 2018. "Emerging nonmetabolic functions of skin fat." *Nature Reviews Endocrinology* 14:163-73.

Gustafson, Birgit, Hammarstedt, Ann, Hedjazifar, Shahram, Smith, Ulf. 2013. "Restricted adipogenesis in hypertrophic obesity: the role of WISP2, WNT, and BMP4." *Diabetes* 62:2997-3004.

György, Bence, Szabo, Tamás G., Pásztói, Maria, Pál, Zsuzsanna, Misják, Petra, Aradi, Borbála, László, Valéria, Pállinger, Éva, Pap, Erna, Kittel, Ágnes, Nagy, Gyögy, Falus, András, Buzás, Edit I. 2011. "Membrane vesicles, current state-of-the-art: emerging role of extracellular vesicles." *Cellular and Molecular Life Sciences* 68:2667-88.

Hysop, Louise, Stojkovic, Miodrag, Armstrong, Lyle, Walter, Theresia, Stojkovic, Petra, Przyborski, Stefan, Herbert, Mary, Murdoch, Alison, Strachan, Tom, Lako, Majlinda. 2005. "Downregulation of NANOG induces differentiation of human embryonic stem cells to extraembryonic lineages." *Stem Cells* 23:1035-43.

Jeppesen, Dennis K., Fenix, Aidan M., Franklin, Jeffrey L., Higginbotham, James N., Zhang, Qin, Zimmerman, Lisa J., Liebler, Daniel C., Ping, Jie, Liu, Qi, Evans, Rachel, Fissell, William H., Patton, James G., Rome, Leonard H., Burnette, Dylan T., Coffey, Robert J. 2019. "Reassessment of Exosome Composition." *Cell* 177:428-45.

Jiang, Nan, Xiang, Lusai, He, Ling, Yang, Guodong, Zheng, Jinxuan, Wang, Chenglin, Zhang, Yimei, Wang, Sainan, Zhou, Yue, Shue, Tzong-Jen, Wu, Jiaqian, Chen, Kenian, Coelho, Paulo G., Tovar, Nicky M., Kim, Shin Hye, Chen, Mo, Zhou, Yan-Heng, Mao, Jeremy J. 2017. "Exosomes mediate epithelium-mesenchyme crosstalk in organ development." *ACS Nano* 11:7736-46.

Jin, Su-Eon and Sung, Jong-Hyuk. 2016. "Hair regeneration using adipose-derived stem cells." *Histology and Histopathology* 31:249-56.

Kimmerling, Kelly A., McQuilling, John P., Staples, Miranda C., Mowry, Katie C. 2018. "Tenocyte cell density, migration, and extracellular matrix deposition with amniotic suspension allograft." *Journal of Orthopaedic Research* 37:412-20.

Kinnaird, T., Stabile, E., Burnett, M. S., Lee, C. W., Barr, S., Fuchs, S., Epstein, S. E. 2004. "Marrow-derived stromal cells express genes encoding a broad spectrum of arteriogenic cytokines and promote in vitro and in vivo arteriogenesis through paracrine mechanisms." *Circulation Research* 94:678-85.

Kitagawa, Tomoko, Matsuda, Ken-Ichi, Inui, Shigeki, Takenaka, Hideya, Katoh, Norito, Itami, Satoshi, Kishimoto, Saburo, Kawata, Mitsuhiro. 2009. "Keratinocyte growth inhibition through the modification of Wnt signaling by androgen in balding dermal papilla cells." *Journal of Clinical Endocrinology & Metabolism* 94:1288-94.

Komiya, Yuko and Habas, Raymond. 2008. "Wnt signal transduction pathways." *Organogenesis* 4:68-75.

Kowal, Joanna, Tkach, Mercedes, Théry, Clotilde. 2014. "Biogenesis and secretion of exosomes." *Current Opinion in Cell Biology* 29:116-25.

Kwack, Mi H., Seo, Chang H., Gangadaran, Prakash, Ahn, Byeong-Cheol, Kim, Moon K., Kim, Jung C., Sung, Young K. 2019. "Exosomes derived from human dermal papilla cells promote hair growth in cultured human hair follicles and augment the hair-inductive capacity of cultured dermal papilla spheres." *Experimental Dermatology* 28:854-71.

L, Praveen Kumar, Kandoi, Sangeetha, Misra, Ranjita, S, Vijayalakshmi, K, Rajagopal, Verma, Rama Shanker. 2019. "The mesenchymal stem cell secretome: A new paradigm towards cell-free therapeutic mode in regenerative medicine." *Cytokine and Growth Factor Reviews* 46:1-9.

Li, Kecheng, Gao, Jinhua, Zhang, Zhidan, Li, Jie, Cha, Pengfei, Liao, Yunjun, Wang, Guan, Lu, Feng. 2013. "Selection of donor site fat grafting and cell isolation." *Aesthetic Plastic Surgery* 37:153-58.

Li, Zheng J., Choi, Hye-In, Choi, Dae-Kyoung, Sohn, Kyung-Cheol, Im, Myung, Seo, Young-Joon, Lee Young-Ho, Lee, Jeung-Hoon, Lee, Young. 2012. "Autologous platelet-rich plasma: A potential therapeutic tool for promoting hair growth." *Dermatologic Surgery* 38:1040-46.

Lichtenberger, Beate M., Mastrogiannaki, Maria, Watt, Fiona M. 2016. "Epidermal β-catenin activation remodels the dermis via paracrine signaling to distinct fibroblast lineages." *Nature Communications* 7:10537.

Lin, Che-Wei, Chen, Yi-Kai, Tang, Kao-Chun, Yang, Kai-Chiang, Cheng, Nai-Chen, Yu, Jiashing. 2018. "Keratin scaffolds with human adipose stem cells: Physical and biological effects toward wound healing." *Journal of Tissue Engineering and Regenerative Medicine* 13:1044-58.

Lin, Wei-hong, Xiang, Li-Jun, Shi, Hong-Xue, Zhang, Jian, Jiang, Li-ping, Cai, Ping-tao, Lin, Zhen-Lang, Lin, Bei-Bei, Huang, Yan, Zhang, Hai-Lin, Fu, Xiao-Bing, Guo, Ding-Jiong, Li, Xiao-Kun, Wang, Xiao-Jie, Xiao, Jian. 2015. "Fibroblast growth factors stimulate hair growth through β-catenin and Shh expression in C57BL/6 mice." *BioMed Research International* 2015:730139.

Liu, Ying, Wang, Haidong, Wang, Juan. 2018. "Exosomes as a novel pathway for regulating development and disease of the skin." *Biomedical Reports* 8:207-24.

Lobb, Richard J., Becker, Melanie, Wen, Shu Wen, Wong, Christina S. F., Wiegmans, Adrian P., Leimgruber, Antoine, Moller, Andreas. 2015. "Optimized exosome isolation protocol for cell culture supernatant and human plasma." *Journal of Extracellular Vesciles* 4:27031.

Lo Celso, Cristina, Prowse, David M., Watt, Fiona M. 2004. "Transient activation of beta-catenin signalling in adult mouse epidermis is sufficient to induce new hair follicles but continuous activation is required to maintain hair follicle tumours." *Development* 131:1787-99.

Lowry, William E., Blanpain Cédric, Nowak Jonathan A., Guasch Geraldine, Lewis Lisa, Fuchs Elaine. 2005. "Defining the impact of beta-catenin/Tcf transactivation on epithelial stem cells." *Genes & Development* 19:1596-611

Mark, Kingston K. L. and Chan, Siu Yuen. 2003. "Epidermal growth factor as a biologic switch in hair growth cycle." *Journal of Biological Chemistry* 278:26120-26.

Marquez-Curtis, Leah A., Janowska-Wieczorek, Anna, McGann, Locksley E., Elliott, Janet A.W. 2015. "Mesenchymal stromal cells derived from various tissues: Biological, clinical and cryopreservation." *Cryobiology* 71:181-97.

Merrill, Bradley J., Gat, Uri, DasGupta, Ramanuj, Fuchs, Elaine. 2001. "Tcf3 and Lef1 regulate lineage differentiation of multipotent stem cells in skin." *Genes & Development* 15:1688-705.

Mittelbrunn, Maria and Sanchez-Madrid, Francisco. 2012. "Intercellular communication: Diverse structures for exchange of genetic information." *Nature Review Molecular and Cell Biology* 13:328-35.

Niknejad, Hassan, Deihim, Tina, Solati-Hashjin, Mehran, Peirovi, Habibollah. 2011. "The effects of preservation procedures on amniotic membrane's ability to serve as a substrate for cultivation of endothelial cells." *Cryobiology* 63:145-51.

Niknejad, Hassan, Peirovi, Habibollah, Jorjanji, Masoumeh, Ahmadiani, Abolhassan, Ghanavi, Jalal, Seifalian, Alexander M. 2008. "Properties of the amniotic membrane for potential use in tissue engineering." *European Cells and Materials* 15:88-99.

Noverina, Rachmawati, Widowati, Wahyu, Ayuningtyas, Wireni, Kurniawan, Dedy, Afifah, Ervi, Laksmitawati, Dian Ratih, Rinendyaputri, Ratih, Rilianawati, Rilianawati, Faried, Ahmad, Bachtiar, Indra, Wirakusumah, Firman Faud. 2019. "Growth factors profile in conditioned medium human adipose tissue-derived mesenchymal stem cells (CH-hATMSCs)." *Clinical Nutrition Experimental* 24:34-44.

Nurden, Alan T. 2011. "Platelets, inflammation and tissue regeneration." *Thrombosis and Haemostasis* 105:S13-S33.

Nyman, Erika, Huss, Fredrik, Nyman, Torbjörn, Junker, Johan, Kratz, Gunnar. 2013. "Hyaluronic acid, an important factor in the wound healing properties of amniotic fluid: *In vitro* studies of re-epithelialisation in human skin wounds." *Journal of Plastic Surgery and Hand Surgery* 47:89-92.

Panero, Alberto J., Hirahara, Alan M., Andersen, Wyatt J., Rothenberg, Joshua, Fierro, Fernando. 2019. "Are amniotic fluid products stem cell therapies?" *The American Journal of Sports Medicine* 47:1230-35.

Park, Junghyun, Kyoung, Jun, Son, Daryeon, Hong, Wonjun, Jang, Jihoon, Yun, Wonjin, Yoon, Byung Sun, Song, Gwonhwa, Kim, In Yong, You, Seungkwon. 2019. "Overexpression of Nanog in amniotic fluid-derived mesenchymal stem cells accelerates dermal papilla cell activity and promotes hair follicle regeneration." *Experimental & Molecular Medicine* 51:72.

Pemberton, Max. 2019. "Why going bald can seriously affect your mental health." *Patient,* March 8. Accessed on July 22, 2019. https://patient.info/news-and-features/can-going-bald-cause-depression.

Peng, Linyi, Jia, Zhuqing, Yin, Xinhua, Zhang, Xin, Liu, Yinan, Chen, Ping, Ma, Kangtao, Zhou, Chunyan. 2008. "Comparative analysis of mesenchymal stem cells from bone marrow, cartilage, and adipose tissue." *Stem Cells and Development* 17:761-73.

Perepelkin, Natasha M. J., Hayward, Kirsten, Mokoena, Tumelo, Bentley, Michael J., Ross-Rodriguez, Lisa U., Marquez-Curtis, Leah, McGann, Locksley E., Holovati, Jelena L., Elliott, Janet A. W. 2015. "Cryopreserved amniotic membrane as transplant allograft: viability and post-transplant outcome." *Cell Tissue Bank* 17:39-50.

Perez-Meza, David, Ziering, Craig, Sforza, Marcos, Krishnan, Ganesh, Ball, Edward, Daniels, Eric. 2017. "Hair follicle growth by stromal vascular fraction-enhanced adipose transplantation into baldness." *Stem Cells and Cloning: Advances and Applications* 10:1-10.

Plikus, Maksim V., Mayer, Julie, de la Cruz, Damon, Baker, Ruth E., Maini, Philip K., Maxson, Robert, Chuong, Cheng-Ming. 2008.

"Cyclic dermal BMP signaling regulates stem cell activation during hair regeneration." *Nature* 451:340-44.

Qi, Hui, Liu, Dan-Ping, Xiao, Da-Wei, Tian, Da-Chuan, Su, Yong-Wei, Jin, Shao-Feng. 2019. "Exosomes derived from mesenchymal stem cells inhibit mitochondrial dysfunction-induced apoptosis of chondrocytes via p38, ERK, Akt pathways." *In Vitro Cellular & Developmental Biology – Animal* 55:203-10.

Rajendran, Ramya Lakshmi, Gangadaran, Prakash, Bak, Soon Sun, Oh, Ji Min, Kalimuthu, Senthilkumar, Lee, Ho Won, Baek, Se Hwan, Zhu, Liya, Sung, Youn Kwan, Jeong, Shin Young, Lee, Sang-Woo, Lee, Jaetae, Ahn, Byeong-Cheol. 2017. "Extracellular vesicles derived from MSCs activates dermal papilla cell *in vitro* and promotes hair follicle conversion from telogen to anagen in mice." *Scientific Reports* 7:15560.

Rivera-Gonzalez, Guillermo C., Shook, Brett A., Andrae, Johanna, Holtrup, Brandon, Bollag, Katherine, Betsholtz, Christer, Rodeheffer, Matthew S., Horsley, Valerie. 2016. "Skin adipocyte stem cell self-renewal is regulated by a PDGFA/Akt signaling axis." *Cell Stem Cell* 19:738-51.

Robinson, Megan J., Cobb, Melanie H. 1997. "Mitogen-activated protein kinase pathways." *Current Opinion in Cell Biology* 9:180-86.

Rong, Xiaoli, Liu, Junzhi, Yao, Xia, Jiang, Tiechao, Wang, Yimin, Xie, Feng. 2019. "Human bone marrow mesenchymal stem cells-derived exosomes alleviate liver fibrosis through the Wnt/β-catenin pathway." *Stem Cell Research & Therapy* 10:98.

Sagaradze, Georgy, Grigorieva, Olga, Nimiritsky, Peter, Basalova, Nataliya, Kalinina, Natalia, Akopyan, Zhanna, Efimenko, Anastasia. 2019. "Conditioned medium from human mesenchymal stromal cells: Towards the clinical translation." *International Journal of Molecular Sciences* 20:1656.

Schmidt, Barbara and Horsley, Valerie. 2012. "Unraveling hair follicle-adipocyte communication." *Experimental Dermatology* 21:827-30.

Seo, Hyung-Sik, Lee, Dong-Jin, Chung, Jae-ho, Lee, Chang-Hyun, Kim, Ha Rim, Kim, Jae Eun, Kim, Byung Joo, Jung, Myeong Ho, Ha, Ki-

Tae, Jeoung, Han-Sol. 2016. "*Hominis Placenta* facilitates hair regrowth by upregulating cellular proliferation and expression of fibroblast growth factor-7." *BMC Complementary & Alternative Medicine* 16:187.

Shin, Hyoseung, Ryu, Hyeong Ho, Kwon, Ohsang, Park, Byung-Soon. 2015. "Clinical use of conditioned media of adipose tissue-derived stem cells in female pattern hair loss: a retrospective case series study." *Pharmacology and Therapeutics* 54:730-35.

Shook, Brett, Gonzalez, Guillermo Rivera, Ebmeier, Sarah, Grisotti, Gabriella, Zwick, Rachel, Horsley, Valerie. 2016. "The role of adipocytes in tissue regeneration and stem cell niches." *Annual Review of Cell and Developmental Biology* 32:609-31.

Tang, Qi Qun and Lane, M. Daniel. 2012. "Adipogenesis: From stem cell to adipocyte." *Annual Review of Biochemistry* 81:715-36.

Tawfik, Abeer Attia and Osman, Mai Abdel Raouf. 2017. "The effect of autologous activated platelet-rich plasma injection on female pattern hair loss: A randomized placebo-controlled study." *Journal of Cosmetic Dermatology* 17:47-53.

Théry, Clotilde, Amigorena, Sebastian, Raposa, Graça, Clayton, Aled. 2006. "Isolation and characterization of exosomes from cell culture supernatants and biological fluids." *Current Protocols in Cell Biology* 30:3.22.1-29.

Tkach, Mercedes and Théry, Clotilde. 2016. "Communication by extracellular vesicles: Where we are and where we need to go." *Cell* 164:1226-32.

Tkach, Mercedes, Kowal, Joanna, Théry, Clotilde. 2017. "Why the need and how to approach the functional diversity of extracellular vesicles." *Philosophical Transactions B* 373:20160479.

Toda, Ayaka, Okabe, Motonori, Yoshida, Toshiko, Nikaido, Toshio. 2007. "The potential of amniotic membrane/amnion-derived cells for regeneration of various tissues." *Journal of Pharmacological Science* 105:215-28.

Tomita, Y., Akiyama, M., Shimizu, H. 2006. "PDGF isoforms induce and maintain anagen phase of murine hair follicles." *Journal of Dermatological Science* 43:105-15.

Tong, Shichao, Zhang, Changqing, Liu, Ji. 2017. "Platelet-rich plasma exhibits beneficial effects for rheumatoid arthritis mice by suppressing inflammatory factors." *Molecular Medicine Reports* 16:4082-88.

Underwood, Mark A., Gilbert, William M., Sherman, Michael P. 2005. "Amniotic fluid: Not just fetal urine anymore." *Journal of Perinatology* 25:341-48.

Van Niel, Guillaume, D'Angelo, Gisela, Raposo, Graça. 2018. "Shedding light on the cell biology of extracellular vesicles." *Nature Reviews Molecular Cell Biology* 19:213-28.

Villarroya-Beltri, Carolina, Baixauli, Francesc, Gutiérrez-Vázquez, Cristina, Sánchez-Madrid, Francisco, Mittelbrunn, María. 2014. *Seminars in Cancer Biology* 28:3-13.

Weger, Nicole and Schlake, Thomas. 2005. "IGF-1 signalling controls the hair growth cycle and the differentiation of hair shafts." *Journal of Investigative Dermatology* 125:873-82.

Werber, Bruce and Martin, Erin. 2013. "A prospective study of 20 foot and ankle wounds treated with cryopreserved amniotic membrane and fluid allograft." *The Journal of Foot & Ankle Surgery* 52:615-21.

Won, Chong Hyun, Yoo, Hyeon Gyeong, Kwon, Oh Sang, Sung, Mi Young, Kang, Yong Jung, Chung, Jin Ho, Park, Byun Soon, Sung, Jong-Hyuk, Kim, Won Serk, Kim, Kyu Han. 2010. "Hair growth promoting effects of adipose tissue-derived stem cells." *Journal of Dermatological Science* 57:134-37.

Yan, Hailong, Gao, Ye, Ding, Qiang, Liu, Jiao, Li, Yan, Jin, Miaohan, Xu, Han, Ma, Sen, Wang, Xiaolong, Zeng, Wenxian, Chen, Yulin. 2019. "Exosomal micro RNAs derived from dermal papilla cells mediate hair follicle stem cell proliferation and differentiation." *International Journal of Biological Sciences* 15:1368-82.

Yang, Jin, Zhao, Shaolin, Yang, Xinling, Zhang, Huanhuan, Zheng, Ping, Wu, Huiyi. 2015. "Inhibition of B-cell apoptosis is mediated through increased expression of Bcl-2 in patients with rheumatoid arthritis." *International Journal of Rheumatic Disease* 19:134-40.

Yoon, Byung Sun, Moon, Jai-Hee, Jun, Eun Kyoung, Kim, Jonggun, Maeng, Isaac, Kim, Jun Sung, Lee, Jung Han, Baik, Cheong Soon, Kim, Aeree, Cho, Kyoung Shik, Lee, Jang Ho, Lee, Hwang Heui, Whang, Kwang Youn, You, Seungkwon. 2010. "Secretory profiles and wound healing effects of human amniotic fluid-derived mesenchymal stem cells." *Stem Cells and Development* 19:887-902.

Zhang, Bing, Tsai, Pai-Chi, Gonzalez-Celeiro, Meryem, Chung, Oliver, Boumard, Benjamin, Perdigoto, Carolina N., Ezhkova, Elean, Hsu, Ya-Chieh. 2016. "Hair follicles' transit-amplifying cells govern concurrent dermal adipocyte production through sonic hedgehog." *Genes & Development* 30:2325-38.

Zhao, Bin, Liu, Jia-Qi, Zheng, Zhao, Zhang, Jun, Wang, Shu-Yue, Han, Shi-Chao, Zhou, Qin, Guan, Hao, Li, Chao, Su, Lin-Lin, Hu, Da-Hai. 2016. "Human amniotic epithelial stem cells promote wound healing by facilitating migration and proliferation of keratinocytes via ERK, JNK, and AKT signaling pathways." *Cell and Tissue Research* 365:85-99.

Zhou, Lijuan, Wang, Han, Jing, Jing, Yu, Lijuan, Wu, Xianjie, Lu, Zhongfa. 2018. "Regulation of hair follicle development by exosomes derived from dermal papilla cells." *Biochemical and Biophysical Research Communications* 500:325-32.

Zhu, Min, Zhengyu, Zhou, Chen, Yan, Schreiber, Ronda, Ransom, John T., Fraser, John K., Hedrick, Marc H., Pinkernell, Kai, Kuo, Hai-Chien. 2010. "Supplementation of fat grafts with adipose-derived regenerative cells improves long-term graft retention." *Annals of Plastic Surgery* 64:222-28.

Zhu, Xishan, Shi, Wei, Tai, Weiping, Liu, Fuquan. 2012. "The comparition of biological characteristics and multilineage differentiation of bone marrow and adipose derived mesenchymal stem cells." *Cell and Tissue Research* 350:277-87.

In: Alopecia
Editor: Pietro Gentile

ISBN: 978-1-53617-008-5
© 2020 Nova Science Publishers, Inc.

Chapter 6

AUTOLOGOUS MICRO-GRAFTS CONTAINING HUMAN HAIR FOLLICLE MESENCHYMAL STEM CELLS (HF-MSCS) FROM SCALP TISSUE: CLINICAL USE IN ANDROGENETIC ALOPECIA

Pietro Gentile[*]

Regenerative Surgery, Plastic and Reconstructive Surgery,
University "Tor Vergata", Rome, Italy

ABSTRACT

Tissue engineering in hair re-growth aims to develop innovative and not invasive procedures to advance the hair re-growt. The use of autologous micro-grafts containing Human Hair Follicle Mesenchymal Stem Cells (HF-MSCs) has not been adequately considered for hair re-growth in patients affected by Androgenic Alopecia. The aim of the

---

[*] Corresponding Author's Email: pietrogentile2004@libero.it.

present chapter is to describe the micro-graft preparation with the possibility to isolate the HF-MSCs. In addition the micro-graft infiltration in the scalp using a mechanical and controlled injections as recently published by the author is described.

This report would also provide a concise review of recent advances in this field confirming that HF-MSCs contained in micro-grafts may represent a safe and viable treatment alternative against hair loss.

ABBREVIATIONS

AD-MSCs	Adipose-derived Mesenchymal Stem Cells
AGA	Androgenic Alopecia
A-PRP	Autologous-Platelet-Rich-Plasma
CAT	Committe for Advanced treatments
CD	Cluster of differentiation
DP	Dermal papilla (DP)
DPCs	Dermal papilla cells
EC	European Parliament
ECM	Extracellular matrix
FGF-7	Fibroblast Growth Factor-7
FT	Fat tissue
GCP	Good Clinical Practices
GFs	Growth Factors
GMP	Good Manufacturing Practices
HC	Hair Count
HD	Hair Density
HF	Hair Follicle
HF-ESCs	Hair Follicle Epithelial Stem Cells
HF-MSCs	Human follicle mesenchymal stem cells
HFs	Hair Follicles
HFSC	Human follicle stem cells
HG	Hair Growth
IGF-1	Insulin like Growth factor-1
KCs	Skin epidermal keratinocytes

Ls	Ludwig scale
NaCl	Saline solution
NHs	Norwood- Hamilton scale
PDGF	Platelet Derived Growth factors
SCs	Stem Cells
SCs	Stem Cells
SPSS	Statistical Package for the Social Sciences
ST	Scalp tissue
SVFs	Stromal vascular Fraction Cells
TA	Targeted Area
VEGF	Vascular endotelial Growth factors

INTRODUCTION

In Androgenic Alopecia (AGA), the miniaturization of the follicles is deteremined by a diminishment of anagen, with an improvement in the percentage of resting hair follicles (HFs), telogen, containing microscopic hairs in a hairless scalp (Paus and Cotsarelis 1999). Moreover, invading lymphocytes and mast cells have been seen around the miniaturizing follicle (Jaworsky, 1992), detailed in the stem cell-rich lump zone (Cotsarelis, 1990).

In hair loss scalp, hair follicle stem cells numbers stay unaltered, though the number of more actively proliferating progenitor cells particularly diminishes (Garza 2011). This proposes going bald scalp either does not have an activator or has an inhibitor of hair follicle (HF) growth.

In a previous study (Gentile 2017) the author showed the use of autologous micro-grafts, reporting mechanical detachment of human hair follicle stem cells (HFSCs) not-expanded got by a slow centrifugation according to minimal manipulation rules, using a CE medical device.

The aim of the present chapter is to describe and evaluate the results in hair re-growth using micro-grafts obtained by the Gentile protocol (Gentile 2019) without the use of CE medical device.

The author reports here, the clinical long-term efficacy of micro-grafts injections and also compared the results obtained with placebo.

This report would also provide a concise review of recent advances in this field.

Additionally, patients' fulfillment and computerized trichogram examination have affirmed the quality of the outcomes.

DATA AND METHODS

AGA Diagnoses must be established performing detailed therapeutic history, clinical examination, blood test and urinalysis, trichoscopic highlights.

The grade of AGA in the selected patients must be estimated according to the Norwood- Hamilton (NHs) for male and Ludwig (Ls) scales for females.

Micro-Graft Preparation According to the "Gentile Protocol"

Autologous micro-grafts of HF-MSCs can be prepared using the "Gentile protocol" (Gentile 2019) (Figure 1A-D and Figure 2A-D), modifying and improving the procedure published previously (Gentile 2017). This protocol represents an innovative clinical approach to obtain autologous micro-grafts through a mechanical fragmentation of different biological tissues (epidermis, dermal, fat tissue, hair, bulb, bulge area) and requires different steps of execution. First step: harvesting of the scalp tissues (30-50 fragments depending by the size of area to treat) with punch biopsy (2mm diameter) (Figure 1A), stored in saline solution and cutting the fragments into strips of 2.0 × 2.0 millimeters (mm) (Figure 1B) collecting and disaggregation of the strips (group of 3 fragments each time) sterilely through a manual splitting perfomed by multiple incisions with scalpel number 11 (Figure 1C) in 1.2mL of saline (NaCl 0,9%) for each 3 fragments with the aim to sort a cell group having a diameter of 80-120 μm; second step: collecting the suspension obtained, average 20ml for 50 fragments disaggregated and fragmented (Figure 1D and Figure 2A), in two 10mL luer-look syringe and centrifugation for 3 minutes at 3000RPM (Figure 2B); 1.5mL of the supernatant was removed for each syringe and 9ml of micro-graft's suspension was obtained; two syringes containing 4,5 ml of micro-graft's suspension were positioned in a mesotherapy gun (Figure 2C); third step: mechanical and controlled infiltration, using 10ml syringes into the selected area of the scalp through a medical device, mesotherapy gun, equipped with a software that allows to schedule the depth of injection, the amount of infiltration per cm^2, with the same angle of inclination (Figure 2D).

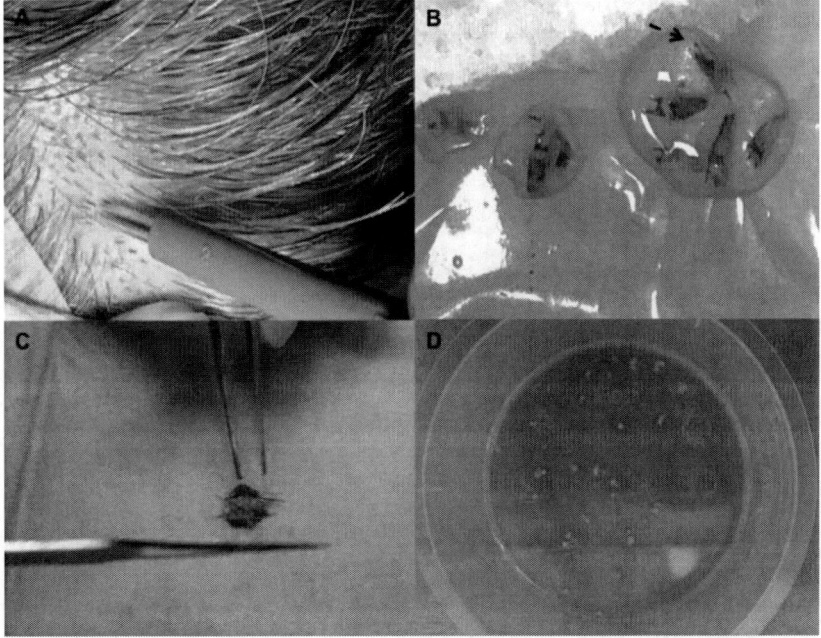

Figure 1. Micro-graft's preparation with "Gentile Protocol" (First and Second steps). (a) Harvesting of the scalp tissues with punch biopsy (2mm diameter). (b) Scalp tissues stored in saline solution. (c) Cutting and splitting of the fragments into strips of 2.0 × 2.0 millimeters (mm) (group of 3 fragments each time) sterilely through a manual splitting perfomed by multiple incisions with scalpel number 11 in 1.2mL of saline for each 3 fragments. (d) Strips splitted and suspension obtained, average 20ml for 50 fragments diaggregated and fragmented.

Micro-Grafts Injections

The scalp must be divided into six different anatomical areas (left frontal area, right frontal area, left parietal area, right parietal area, left vertex area and right vertex area); anesthesia (local or potentially fundamental) is not necessary. The micro-grafts suspension inter-follicular infusions (0.2 mL/cm^2) must be injected to targeted area (TA) at 5 mm depth utilizing a mesotherapy medical device outfitted with a 10 mL syringe luer-lock with needle 30-gauge, in three sessions spaced 45 days apart.

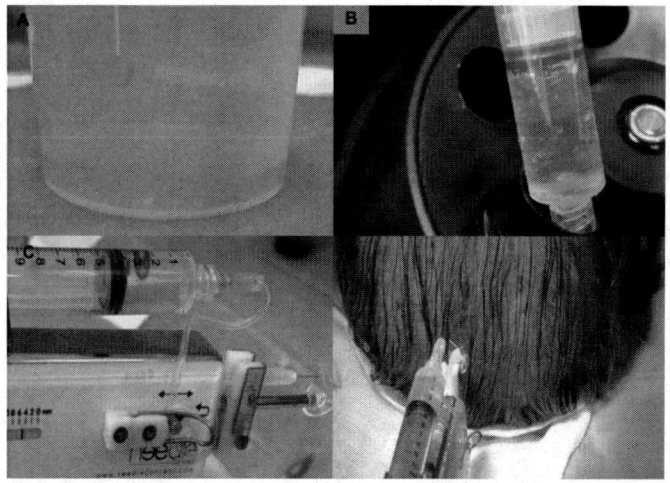

Figure 2. Micro-graft's preparation with "Gentile Protocol" (Third step). (a) 20ml of suspension containing strips splitted. (b) Collecting the suspension obtained, in two 10mL luer-look syringe and centrifugation for 3 minutes at 3000RPM. (c) Two syringes containing 4,5 ml of micro-graft's suspension were positioned in a mesotherapy gun. (d) Mechanical and controlled infiltration, using 10ml syringes into the selected area of the scalp through a mesotherapy gun.

Clinical Assessment of Hair Growth

Assessment of hair growth (HG) may be evaluated in different weeks (Ws) after the treatment, that could be summarized in four phases: T0

(Figure 3A,B), before the first infusion (Figures 4A, 5A), T1 - 3 Ws, T2 - 9 Ws (Figure 4B), T3 - 16 Ws, T4 - 23 Ws (Figure 4C), T5 - 58 Ws after the last treatment (Figures 3C,D, 4D, 5B).

The impacts of micro-grafts' suspension on HG must be evaluated using photography (same position, same contrast, same light), the physician's and patient's global evaluation scale, and standardized phototrichograms.

In all partecipants, TA has been marked with a semi-permanent tattoo for the subsequent trichogram.

Phototrichograms (Figure 3A-D) were performed in all TA using Fotofinder videoepiluminescence systems in combination with the Trichoscan digital image analysis. TrichoScan evaluate hairs per $0.65cm^2$ described as hair count (HC), hairs per cm^2 described as hair density (HD), hair thickness (HT), anagen-to-telogen ratio, and vellus hair-to-terminal hair ratio. All hairs with a thickness > 40 μm are categorized as terminal hairs while those with lesser diameter are categorized as vellus hairs.

Micro-Needling Rules in Hair Re-Growth

Stoll et al. (Stoll 2015) suggested in a pre-clinical model, that superficial mechanical trauma of the skin produced by micro-needling injections would induce long-term hair re-growth. In this study, five Ws after micro-needling injections, hair re-growth started, followed by a hyperpigmentation reduction. 12 Ws later it was reported a 90% improvement in coat coverage at previously thinning areas. 12 months later, coat conditions remained stable (Stoll 2015).

As reported by Ferting et al. (Ferting 2018) in a clinical model review, the micro-needling injections is a not invasive procedure in which very fine needles are rolled over the skin to puncture the stratum corneum, inducing collagen production, angiogenesis and growth factors release. The micro-needling procedure has been tested in a great range of dermatologic pathologies as AGA and alopecia areata (Ferting 2018).

Micro-Grafts Procedures: Enzymatic Digestion versus Mechanical Disaggregaion

HF-MSCs can be isolated by enzymatic digestion or mechanical disaggregation. In the first technique, the scalp fragment is reaped sterilely, processed on proper catalysts, and after that, the resulting cell solutions are seeded in culture dishes containing a unique medium supplemented with vital added substances, and afterward incubated. At long last, the subsequent colonies are sub-cultured before conversion and the cells are fortified to differentiate (Gentile 2017; Zhang, 2013; Yu 2006). According to the European rules (EC n. 1394/2007) and European Medicine Agency (EMA)/Committee for Advanced Treatments (CAT) recommendations (EMA/CAT/600280/2010 Rev 1), it is possible to perform a substantial manipulation of cells expansion in culture and re-injection of the expanded cellular suspension obtained only through Good Manufacturing Practices (GMP) laboratories with Clinical Trial authorized by a Health Ministry.

In fact, the suspension of cells expanded after substantial manipulation is considered an advanced therapy medicinal product. On the other hand, a cellular suspension obtained by enzymatic digestion without cells expansion in culture (only cells isolation), or by mechanical fragmentation, are not considered substantial manipulation in that biological characteristics, physiological functions, or structural properties relevant for the intended clinical use are not altered and in addition they must contain cells that are intended to be used for the same essential function(s) in the recipient area and the donor area. The EMA/CAT considers that the products obtained through this modality of preparation does not fall within the definition of an advanced therapy medicinal product, as provided in Article 2 of Regulation (EC) 1394/2007. In addition, enzymatic digestion procedures have longer preparation times and higher costs. For these reasons, the mechanical fragmentation procedure was preferred to cell expansion or enzymatic digestion procedures.

In the second technique, autologous micro-grafts containing HF-MSCs can be isolated by the "Gentile procedure" in which the scalp is dealt with as some other connective tissue subjected to grafts, with a period of collection and a period of mechanical disaggregation of the tissue without controlling the grid. The "Gentile procedure" can be performed using a medical device, as previously reported (Gentile 2017) or without (Gentile 2019), through a procedure of scalp tissues' splitting producing a great many practical micro-grafts and filters them with a cut-off size of 80–140 microns, to advance the releasing of old separated cells and the improvement of youthful ancestor cells contained inside the scalp tissue (Gentile 2017; Zhang, 2013; Yu 2006; Cotsarelis 1990).

HF-MSCs Identity

HF-MSCs exhibited surface markers of bone marrow mesenchymal stem cells, as shown by positive staining for CD44, CD73, CD90, and CD105, and they also displayed trilineage differentiation potentials into adipocytes, chondrocytes, and osteoblasts by cytochemistry and qRT-PCR (Zhang, 2013).

The human HFs bulge is also an important niche for keratinocyte stem cells and epithelial stem cells (ESCs) (Yu 2006). Positive markers for bulge cells included CD200, follistatin, PHLDA1, and frizzled homolog 1, while CD34, CD24, CD71, and CD146 were preferentially expressed by non-bulge keratinocytes, as reported by Ohyama et al. (Yu 2006).

In addition, CD200+ cells (CD200hiCD24loCD34loCD71loCD146lo) obtained from hair follicle suspensions demonstrated high colony-forming effciency in clonogenic assays, indicating successful enrichment of living human bulge stem cells (Yu 2006).

For ST, in a previous research conducted by Gentile et al. (Gentile 2017), it was tuning a procedure to collect HFSCs with minimal manipulation based on the centrifugation of scalp's fragments obtained by punch biopsy, without cellular extension or culture. In this procedure, we succeeded in cell counting and identifying of CD44+ HF-MSCs and the CD200+ HF-ESCs, according to previously reported studies (Zhang, 2013).

In patients affected by AGA with scalp presenting hair loss, the HFSCs numbers were reported to remain unaltered; however, the quantity of the more effectively multiplying progenitors cells significantly decreases (Garza 2011).

However, the reconstitution of a completely sorted out and utilitarian HF from separated cells propagated under characterized tissue culture conditions is a test as yet pending in tissue engineering (Balañá 2015). HFs contains a niche for grown-up stem cells represented by lump, containing epithelial and melanocytic stem cells (Yu 2006).

SCs in the hair lump, an obviously differentiated structure inside the lower permanent portion of HFs, can generate the interfollicular epidermis, HF structures, and sebaceous glands (Cotsarelis 1990; Tumbar 2004). The lump ESCs can likewise reconstitute in a simulated *in vivo* framework to a new HF (Morris 2004; Taylor 2000).

HF-MSCs Potential

Yu et al. (Yu 2006) demonstrated that human HFs contains a stem cell populace that may be separated into the neuron, smooth muscle cell, and melanocyte heredities in induction medium. Their information demonstrates that Oct4-positive cells are available in human skin, and the majority of them are situated in the HFs *in vivo*. Oct4 has a place with the family of POU-domain transcription factors that are regularly communicated in pluripotent cells of the developing embryo and mediate pluripotency (Pesce 2001). Each mature HF is a regenerating framework, which physiologically experiences cycles of growth (anagen), relapse (catagen), and rest (telogen) various times in grown-up's life (Alonso and Fuchs 2006). In catagen, HFSCs are kept up in the lump. At that point, the resting follicle re-enters anagen (regeneration) when legitimate molecular signals are given. Amid late telogen to early anagen change, signals from the Dermal Papilla (DP) stimulate the hair germ and quiescent lump stem cells to wind up activated (Greco 2009).

Numerous paracrine factors are engaged with this crosstalk at various hair cycle stages and some signaling pathways have been implicated (Blanpain 2004; Botchkarev 2003; Roh, 2004). In anagen, SCs in the lump offer ascent to hair germs, at that point the transient increasing cells in the grid of the new follicle proliferate quickly to frame another hair filament (Hsu 2001).

As a matter of fact, the authors feel the need to better know in which stage is necessary to act. Regeneration of HFs was likewise seen in people (Reynolds 1999) when dermal sheath tissue was utilized, which was adequate to regenerate additionally the DP structure. After implantation, the whisker DP was equipped for promoting HF regeneration holding the data to decide hair fiber type and follicle size (Jahoda 1992). Grafting of dermal-inductive tissue was restricted by the way that it was impractical to produce more HFs than the one obtained from the donor tissues. To defeat this constraint diverse methodologies and exploratory models utilizing freshly or cultured isolated cells from both dermal and dermal/epidermal origin were tried. The vast majority of them included neonatal and embryonic murine cells.

Balañá ME et al. (Balañá 2015) in a pre-clinical model, created a dermal-epidermal skin substitute by seeding cultured human derived HF-ESCs and DPCs, in an acellular dermal grid. This product were grafted into a wound produced on bare mice skin and fourteen days later, in the treated area, histological structures reminiscent of a great range of phases of embryonic HF improvement was identified, demonstrating concentric cellular layers of human origin and expressed k6hf, keratin in epithelial cells of the companion layer. The results obtained suggested that both epithelial and dermal cultured cells from the grown-up human scalp in a dermal scaffold could create *in vivo* structures that reiterate embryonic hair improvement.

Kalabusheva et al. (Kalabusheva 2017) aimed to build up a simulated HF germ, through the combining of post-natal human DPCs and skin epidermal keratinocytes (KCs) in a hanging drop culture. Blended HF germ-like structures showed the start of epithelial-mesenchymal collaboration, including WNT pathway enactment and expression of follicular markers. It was examined the impact of DP cell niche components including dissolvable components and extracellular matrix (ECM) molecules during the time spent on the organoid assembling and growth. The outcomes obtained showed that soluble components had little impact on HF germ generation and Ki67+ cell score inside the organoids despite the fact that BMP6 and VD3 kept up effectively the DP character in the monolayer culture. Talavera-Adame et al. (Talavera-Adame 2017) revealed the biomolecular pathway involved in a cellular therapy.

Specifically, It has been additionally demonstrated that Wnt/β-catenin signaling is necessary for the growth and upkeep of DPCs (Tsai 2014; Huelsken 2001). The increment of Wnt signaling in DPCs evidently is one of the principal factors that enhance HG (Tsai 2014).

Festa et al. (Festa 2011) detailed that adipocyte progenitors cells bolster the SCs niche and help conduct the complex HG cycle. This approach aimed to regenerate HFs is fascinating and raises the likelihood that one can conduct or reestablish the hair cycle in the thinning by stimulating the niche with autologous fat improved with stromal cells.

Along these lines, Perez-Meza D et al. (Perez-Meza 2017) detailed the safety, tolerability, and quantitative, in patients with hereditary thinning treated with sub-cutaneous scalp infusion of advanced FT. The discoveries propose that scalp stem cell-enriched fat grafting may represent a promising elective way to deal with treating hair loss in people.

Fukuoka et al. (Fukuoka 2015) reported a mean increment of 29 ± 4.1 hairs in male patients and 15.6 ± 4.2 hairs in female treated with fat-derived stem cell-conditioned medium infusion.

RESULTS

Clinical and Trichoscopic Results

In a study submitted by the author (Data not published at the time of the present chapter) the results obtained displayed an improvement in the mean HC at T5 after 58 weeks (58 weeks vs. 0 weeks) of 18.0 hairs in the

TA (Figure 3C,D) compared with baseline (Figure 3A,B), while the control area (CA) displayed a mean decrease of 1.1 hairs (control vs. treatment: $p < .0001$). Accordingly, a mean increase in total HD of 23.3 hairs per cm^2 (Figure 3C,D) compared with baseline (Figure 3A,B; Figures 4A, 5A) was observed at T5 (Figure 4D and Figure 5B), and the CA displayed a mean decrease of 0.7 hairs per cm^2 (control vs. treatment: $p < .0001$).

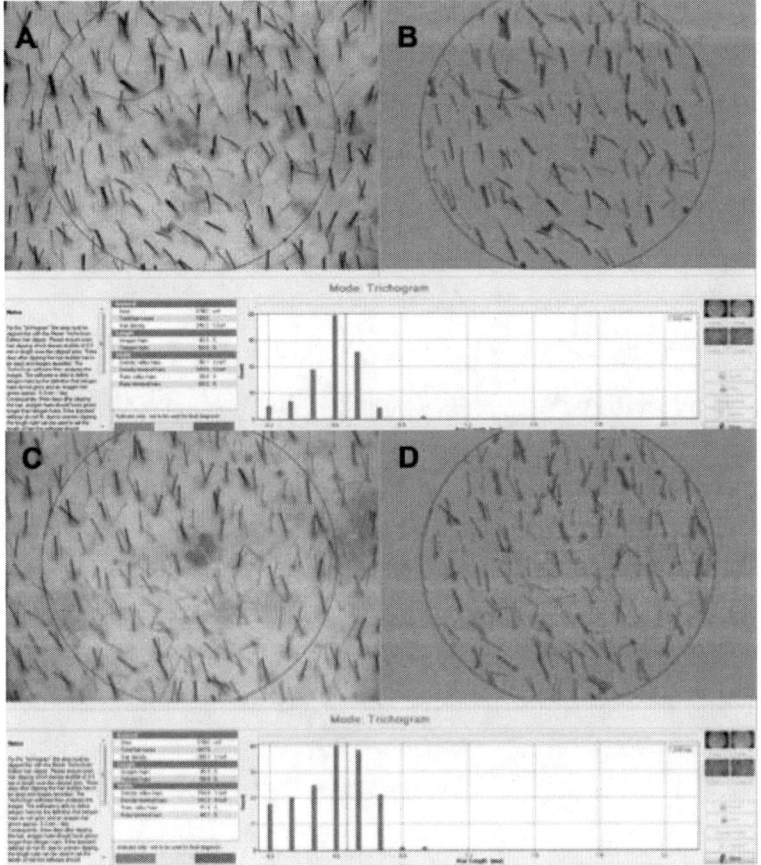

Figure 3. Trichoscan analysis performed by Fotofinder in non-smoker 41-year-old male with AGA, stage 3-Vertex according to NHs, showed in Figure 4. (a, b) At T0 pre-operative HC was 72.2 hairs per 0.65 cm^2; HD was 97.5 hairs per cm^2; and proportions of anagen and telogen hairs were 59.0% and 41.4%, respectively. (c, d) At T5 postoperative HC was 90.5 hairs per 0.65 cm^2; HD was 122.8 hairs per cm^2; and proportions of anagen and telogen hairs were 48.6% and 51.7%, respectively.

There were no statistically significant differences in vellus HD between the TA and the CA at T5. Following 26 months, 6 patients detailed dynamic hair loss. Those six patients were re-treated.

In a study published by the author (Gentile 2019), 23 weeks after the last treatment with micro-graft injection, the mean hair density increments were 33% ± 7.5% over baseline values for the treated region and less than 1% increment for the region infused with saline. 44 weeks after the last treatment, the main hair density increments reported by phototrichograms were 27% ± 3.5% over baseline values for the treated region and not more than a 0.7% increment in hair density for the placebo region.

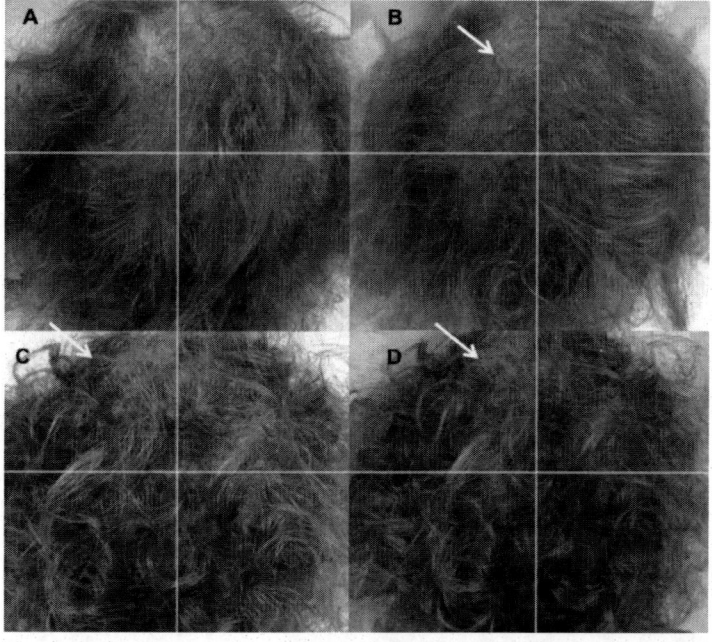

Figure 4. Non-smoker 38-year-old female affected by AGA classified in stage 2 according to Ls. (a) Pre-operative image at T0 with thinning localized to the frontal and parietal areas; (b) Post-perative image at T2 (9 Ws later the last treatment); the arrow indicate the left parietal area treated with two micro-grafts injections with increase of HD vs. right parietal area treated with placebo. (c) Post-perative image at T4 (23 Ws later the last treatment); the arrow indicate again the same area with increase of HD. (d) Post-perative image at T5 (58 Ws later the last treatment); the arrow indicate the final result obtained.

Relapse of hair loss was not assessed in treated patients until a year after the last injection. In the following 16 months, 3 patients detailed dynamic hair loss. Those three patients were re-treated.

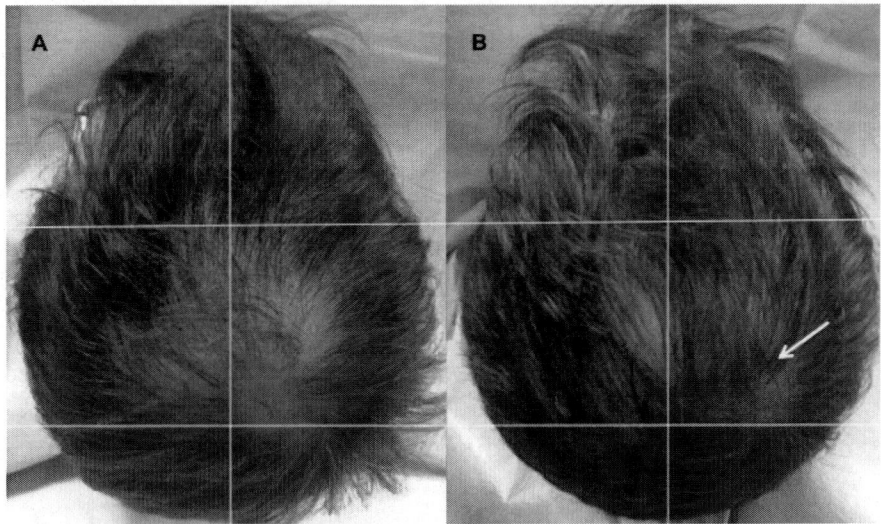

Figure 5. Non-smoker 41-year-old male with AGA classified in stage 3-Vertex according to NHs. (a) Pre-operative image at T0 with thinning localized to the vertex, parietal, temporal and frontal areas; (b) The arrow indicate the post-operative situation of the scalp at T5 after 58 Ws later the last treatment with improvement of HD in the vertex right area treated with two micro-grafts injections vs. baseline situation in the same area and vs vertex left area treated with placebo.

CONCLUSION

The information reported in this chapter obviously highlights the constructive effects of HF-MSCs based on micro-grafts infusions on AGA without major side effects. Compared with previous work published in 2017 (Gentile 2017), the "Gentile procedure" (Gentile 2019) showed better results in term of clinical and trichoscopic outcomes. Micro-grafts containing HF-MSCs may serve as a safe and effective treatment option against hair loss even if more extensive controlled studies are needed to strengthen these results.

REFERENCES

Alonso, L. & Fuchs, E. (2006). The hair cycle. *J Cell Sci.*, *119*, 391-393.

Balañá, M. E., Charreau, H. E. & Leirós, G. J. (2015). Epidermal stem cells and skin tissue engineering in hair follicle regeneration. *World J Stem Cells.*, *26*, 7, 711-27.

Blanpain, C., Lowry, W. E., Geoghegan, A., Polak, L. & Fuchs, E. (2004). Self-renewal, multipotency, and the existence of two cell populations within an epithelial stem cell niche. *Cell.*, *118*, 635-648.

Botchkarev, V. A. & Kishimoto, J. (2003). Molecular control of epithelial-mesenchymal interactions during hair follicle cycling. *J Investig Dermatol Symp Proc.*, *8*, 46-55.

Cotsarelis, G., Sun, T. T. & Lavker, R. M. (1990). Label-retaining cells reside in the bulge area of pilosebaceous unit: Implications for follicular stem cells, hair cycle, and skin carcinogenesis. *Cell*, *61*, 1329–1337.

Fertig, R. M., Gamret, A. C., Cervantes, J. & Tosti, A. (2018). Microneedling for the treatment of hair loss?, *J Eur Acad Dermatol Venereol.*, *32*, 4, 564-569.

Festa, E., Fretz, J., Berry, A., Schmidt, B., Rodeheffer, M., Horowitz, M. & Horsley, V. (2011). Adipocyte lineage cells contribute to the skin stem cell niche to drive hair cycling. *Cell.*, *146*, 761–771.

Fukuoka, H. & Suga, H. (2015). Hair Regeneration Treatment Using Adipose-Derived Stem Cell Conditioned Medium: Follow-up With Trichograms," *Eplasty.*, *15*, e10.

Huelsken, J., Vogel, R., Erdmann, B., Cotsarelis, G. & Birchmeier, W. (2001). Beta-Catenin controls hair follicle morphogenesis and stem cell differentiation in the skin. *Cell.*, *105*, 4, 533–545.

Garza, L. A., Yang, C. C., Zhao, T., Blatt, H. B., Lee, M., He, H., Stanton, D. C., Carrasco, L., Spiegel, J. H., Tobias, J. W. & Cotsarelis, G.

(2011). Bald scalp in men with androgenetic alopecia retains hair follicle stem cells but lacks CD200-rich and CD34-positive hair follicle progenitor cells. *J Clin Invest.*, *121*, 613– 622.

Gentile, P., Scioli, M. G., Bielli, A., Orlandi, A. & Cervelli, V. (2017). Stem cells from human hair follicles: first mechanical isolation for immediate autologous clinical use in androgenetic alopecia and hair loss. *Stem Cell Investig.*, *4*, 58.

Gentile, P. (2019). Autologous Cellular Method Using Micrografts of Human Adipose Tissue Derived Follicle Stem Cells in Androgenic Alopecia. *Int J Mol Sci.*, *13*, 20(14).

Greco, V., Chen, T. & Rendl, M. (2009). A two-step mechanism for stem cell activation during hair regeneration. *Cell Stem Cell.*, *4*, 155-169.

Hsu, Y. C., Pasolli, H. A. & Fuchs, E. (2001). Dynamics between stem cells, niche, and progeny in the hair follicle. *Cell*, vol. *144*, 92-105.

Jahoda, C. A. (1992) Induction of follicle formation and hair growth by vibrissa dermal papillae implanted into rat ear wounds: vibrissa-type fibres are specified. *Development.*, *115*, 1103-1109.

Jaworsky, C., Kligman, A. M. & Murphy, G. F. (1992) Characterization of inflammatory infiltrates in male pattern alopecia: Implications for pathogenesis. *Br J Dermatol.*, *127*, 239–246.

Kalabusheva, E., Terskikh, V. & Vorotelyak, E. (2017). Hair Germ Model *In Vitro* via Human Postnatal Keratinocyte-Dermal Papilla Interactions: Impact of Hyaluronic Acid. *Stem Cells Int.*, 2017, 2017.

Morris, R. J., Liu, Y., Marles, L., Yang, Z., Trempus, C., Li, S., Lin, J. S., Sawicki, J. A. & Cotsarelis, G. (2004). Capturing and profiling adult hair follicle stem cells. *Nat Biotechnol*, *22*, 411–417.

Paus, R. & Cotsarelis, G. (1999). The biology of hair follicles. *N Engl J Med.*, *341*, 491–497.

Pesce, M. & Scholer, H. R. (2001). Oct-4: gatekeeper in the beginnings of mammalian development. *Stem Cells*, *19*, 271–278.

Perez-Meza, D., Ziering, C., Sforza, M., Krishnan, G., Ball, E. & Daniels, E. (2017). Hair follicle growth by stromal vascular fraction-enhanced adipose transplantation in baldness. *Stem Cells Cloning*, *10*, 1-10.

Reynolds, A. J., Lawrence, C., Cserhalmi-Friedman, P. B., Christiano, A. M. & Jahoda, C. A. (1999). Trans-gender induction of hair follicles. *Nature.*, *402*, 33-34.

Roh, C., Tao, Q. & Lyle, S. (2004). Dermal papilla-induced hair differentiation of adult epithelial stem cells from human skin. *Physiol Genomics.*, *19*, 207-217.

Stoll, S., Dietlin, C. & Nett-Mettler, C. S. (2015). Microneedling as a successful treatment for alopecia X in two Pomeranian siblings. *Vet Dermatol.*, *26*, 5, 387-90.

Talavera-Adame, D., Newman, D. & Newman, N. (2017). Conventional and novel stem cell based therapies for androgenic alopecia. *Stem Cells Cloning.*, *10*, 11-19.

Taylor, G., Lehrer, M. S., Jensen, P. J., Sun, T. T. & Lavker, R. M. (2000). Involvement of follicular stem cells in forming not only the follicle but also the epidermis. *Cell.*, *102*, 451–461.

Tsai, S. Y., Sennett, R. & Rezza, A. (2014). Wnt/β-catenin signaling in dermal condensates is required for hair follicle formation. *Dev Biol.*, *385*, 2, 179–188.

Tumbar, T., Guasch, G., Greco, V., Blanpain, C., Lowry, W. E., Rendl, M. & Fuchs, E. (2004). Defining the epithelial stem cell niche in skin. *Science.*, *303*, 359 –363.

Yu, H., Fang, D., Kumar, S. M., Li, l., Nguyen, T. K., Acs, G., Herlyn, M. & Xu, X. (2006). Isolation of a novel population of multipotent adult stem cells from human hair follicles. *Am J Pathol.*, *168*, 1879-88.

Zhang, X., Wang, Y., Gao, Y., Liu, X., Bai, T., Li, M., Li, L., Chi, G., Xu, H., Liu, F., Liu, J. Y. & Li, Y. (2013). Maintenance of high proliferation and multipotent potential of human hair follicle-derived mesenchymal stem cells by growth factors. *Int J Mol Med*, *31*, 913-21.

In: Alopecia
Editor: Pietro Gentile

ISBN: 978-1-53617-008-5
© 2020 Nova Science Publishers, Inc.

Chapter 7

PLATELET RICH PLASMA: CLINICAL USE IN ANDROGENETIC ALOPECIA AND BIOMOLECULAR PATHWAY ANALYSIS

Pietro Gentile[*]

Regenerative Surgery, Plastic and Reconstructive Surgery,
University "Tor Vergata", Rome, Italy

ABSTRACT

Platelet-rich plasma (PRP) has emerged as a new treatment modality in regenerative medicine, and preliminary evidence suggests that it might have a beneficial role in Androgentic Alopecia (AGA). The safety and clinical efficacy of autologous PRP injections for pattern hair loss were investigated in the last 10 years in randomized, placebo-controlled, half-head group study to compare the hair re-growth with PRP versus placebo. No side effects were reported during treatment.

---

[*] Corresponding Author's Email: pietrogentile2004@libero.it.

The aim of the present chapter is to describe the PRP preparation with the possibility to analyze growth factors and biomolecular pathway. In addition it is described the PRP infiltration in the scalp using a mechanical and controlled injections as recently published by the author.

This report would also provide a concise review of recent advances in this field confirming that PRP may represent a safe and viable treatment alternative against hair loss.

INTRODUCTION

A number of products have been proposed as hair-loss therapies. Drug therapies specifically approved by the U.S. Food and Drug Administration (FDA) for treating Androgenetic Alopecia (AGA) are limited to Minoxidil and Finasteride.

Both can be used alone or combined (Gkini 2014). The role of PRP for the treatment of AGA and Alopecia Areata has been demonstrated in old important reports (Li 2012; Khatu 2014; Trink 2013). Recently, the author published many studies focused on clinical and instrumental evaluation of the PRP effects in patients affected by AGA (Gentile 2015; Gentile 2017; Gentile 2019). In addition, the author, described for the first time, the necessity to perform a mechanical and controlled injection of PRP in the scalp using a mesotherapy gun (Gentile 2017; Gentile 2018). Also the biomolecular pathway analysis was perfomed showing the action of growth factors contained in PRP in hair re-growth (Gentile and Garcovich 2019).

As known, the activation of platelet alpha-granules releases numerous growth factors, including transforming growth factor (TGF), plateletderived growth factor (PDGF),vascular endothelial growth factor (VEGF), epidermal growth factor (EGF), insulin-like growth factor, and interleukin-1 (Khatu 2014). It is suggested that growth factors released from platelets may act on stem cells in the bulge area of the follicles, stimulating the development of new follicles and promoting angiogenesis (Khatu 2014). In the bulge area, primitive stem cells of ectodermal origin are found, giving origin to epidermal cells and sebaceous glands. In matrix, germinative cells of mesenchymal origin are found at the dermal papilla. Interactions between these two kinds of cells as well as with binding growth factors (PDGF, TGF-b, andVEGF) activate the proliferative phase of the hair, giving rise to the future follicular unit (Gkini 2014). For these reasons, Gkini et al. (Gkini 2014) and Khatu et al. (Khatu, 2014) have reported in two different works that PRP could serve as a potential treatment for AGA.

PRP has been reported to induce the proliferation of dermal papilla cells by up regulating fibroblast growth factor7 (FGF-7) and beta-catenin, as well as extracellular signal-related kinase (ERK) and Akt signaling ((Li, 2012). The aim of the present chapter is to describe the injections and PRP preparation with the use of CE medical device, evaluating the results in hair re-growth using PRP obtained by autologous blood without cryopreservation. The author report here, the clinical long-term efficacy of PRP injections and compared also the results obtained with placebo. This report would also provide a concise review of recent advances in this field.

Additionally, patients' fulfillment and computerized trichogram examination have affirmed the quality of the outcomes.

DATA AND METHODS

AGA Diagnoses must be established performing detailed therapeutic history, clinical examination, blood test and urinalysis, trichoscopic highlights.

The grade of AGA in the selected patients must be estimated according to the Norwood- Hamilton (NHs) for male and Ludwig (Ls) scales for females.

Platelet Rich Plasma European Rules

Autologous Platelet rich plasma can be prepared using a small volume of blood (9mL – 55mL) according to the European and Italian rules represented by Regulation n. 1394/2007 of the European Parliament (EC) and by the Reflection Paper on characterization of cutting edge treatment medicinal products draft concurred 20 June 2014 EMA/CAT/600280/2010 Rev. 1 Committee for Advanced treatments (CAT) in which the autologous use in one step surgery, minimal manipulation, omofunctional use "used for an indistinguishable fundamental capacity in the beneficiary as in the donor", manipulation with gadgets in aseptic conditions, are conditions that do not require Good Manufacturing Practices (GMP) rules for processing, Good Clinical Practices (GCP) for the clinical application and the ethical Committeee endorsement. PRP preparation must be performed respecting in Italy "Decree of the blood, 2 Novemeber 2015", dispoisitions related to quality and safety parameters of blood and emocomponents.

Platelet Rich Plasma: Different Types of Preparation

The number of papers published on PRP is considerable, but the results are often contradictory. The authors thinking that it is not possible to speak about PRP in general, but it is better to identify different types of PRP preparations depending on their cell content and fibrin architecture. On this way it is possible to identify:

1. Leukocyte-poor PRP (LP-PRP) or Pure Platelet-Rich Plasma (P-PRP). Suspension without leukocytes and with a low-density fibrin network after activation;
2. PRP and Leukocyte (L-PRP). Suspensions with leukocytes and a low densities fibrin network after activation (the largest number of commercial kit);
3. Leukocyte- poor platelet-rich fibrin (LP-PRF) or pure platelet-rich fibrin (P-PRF). Suspensions without leukocytes and a high-density fibrin network.
4. Leukocytes and platelet rich fibrin (L-PRF) or second generations PRP products are preparations with leukocytes and a high-density fibrin network.

As reported, there are too many protocols for preparation of PRP depending on the different time and RPM or G-force used, the platelets number, the availability of growth factors and chemokines. There is also a wide biological (between patients) and temporal (day to day) variation (Gentile 2019). So, it is difficult to assess which kit for PRP preparation is better and which is worse.

Different PRP products might be more or less appropriate to treat different kinds of Alopecia.

Platelet Rich Plasma Preparation: Activated or not Activated?

In hair loss treatment, differences were found when PRP therapies were performed with CE medical device of activated autologous PRP (AA-PRP) in place of non-activated A-PRP.

In the treatment of hair loss, topical use of AA-PRP to harvested follicles prior to implantation has already been shown to increase their survival rate by 15% (Uebel 2006).

Moreover, patients treated with calcium gluconate-activated PRP exhibit increased hair density three months post-surgery with terminal hair density (diameter > 40μm) increasing by 19% during that time.

These findings were confirmed in a study following AGA patients treated with calcium-activated PRP over the course of one year (Gentile 2017).

The growth factors obtained by the degranulation of the alpha-granules have been shown to stimulate hair re-growth. In detail, insulin-like growth factor-1 (IGF-1) stimulates proliferation of cycling Ki67+ basal keratinocytes, while transforming growth factor β1 (TGF-β1) protects the proliferative potential of basal keratinocytes by inhibiting cell growth and terminal differentiation (Gentile 2015, Gentile 2017, Gentile and Garcovich 2019). Platelet-derived growth factor AA (PDGF-AA) increase the hair inductive activity of DPCs when applied in combination with fibroblast growth factor 2 (FGF-2) (Gentile 2015, Gentile 2017, Gentile and Garcovich 2019). Vascular endothelial growth factor (VEGF) stimulates angiogenesis, and PDGF-BB is a potent chemo-attractant for wound macrophages and fibroblasts and stimulates these cells to release endogenous growth factors, including TGF-β1, that promote new collagen synthesis (Gentile 2015, Gentile 2017, Gentile and Garcovich 2019).

Dermal papilla cells (DPCs) harvested from human scalp have shown increased proliferation, increased Bcl-2 and FGF-7 levels, activated ERK and Akt proteins, and up-regulation of β-catenin when cultured in an activated PRP-supplemented growth medium (Gentile 2015, Gentile 2017, Gentile and Garcovich 2019). Since each of these factors positively influences hair re-growth through cellular proliferation to prolong the anagen phase (FGF-7), inducing cell growth (ERK activation), stimulating hair follicle development (β-catenin), and suppressing apoptotic cues (Bcl-2 release and Akt activation) (Gentile 2015, Gentile 2017, Gentile and Garcovich 2019).

Human scalp affected by AGA injected with PRP should display marked increases in cellular activity. Indeed, histological examination of A-PRP and AA-PRP treated scalp from our previous works (Gentile 2015, Gentile 2017, Gentile and Garcovich 2019) provides such clinical evidence.

In both patient populations, the authors observed improvement in the number of follicular bulge cells and follicles, epidermal thickening, improved vascularization, and a higher number of Ki67+ basal keratinocytes in PRP-treated scalp tissue compared with placebo.

Platelet Rich Plasma Preparation Using CE Medical Device: Experience of the Author

PRP was prepared in all caese, respecting the European and Italian rules.

All patients signed the informed consent. For this reason PRP was obtained from a small volume of autologous blood (9mL – 55mL) using different CE medical device with protocol tested and approved by the transfusional service. As published, the author reported his own experience using the Cascade-Selphyl-Esforax system (Aesthetic Factors, LLC, Wayne, NJ, http://www.selphyl.com) (Activated PRP –AA-PRP-) (Figure 1), with modifications, and the C-punt system (Biomed Device, Modena, Itlay, http://www.biomeddevice.it) (Not- Activated PRP -A-PRP-) (Figure 2) (Gentile 2015).

Briefly, blood was taken from a peripheral vein using sodium citrate as an anticoagulant. The current systems for preparing platelet concentrations use various centrifuges (in the Cascade-Selphyl-Esforax procedure, we used 1,100g for 10 minutes; in C-Punt system,we used 1,200rpm for 10 minutes).

Although the method of preparation is not selective and may include leukocytes, the final aim is to obtain a platelet pellet.

Growth factors are secreted only once platelet activation begins, which, in turn, is stimulated by calcium (Ca2+).

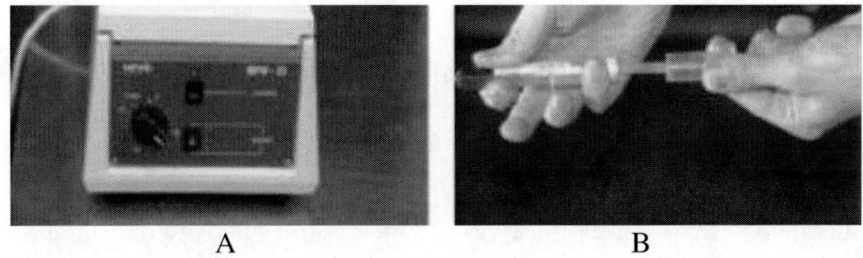

Figure 1. Platelet rich plasma preparation with Cascade procedure (A) Centrifuge. (B) activation with Ca2+.

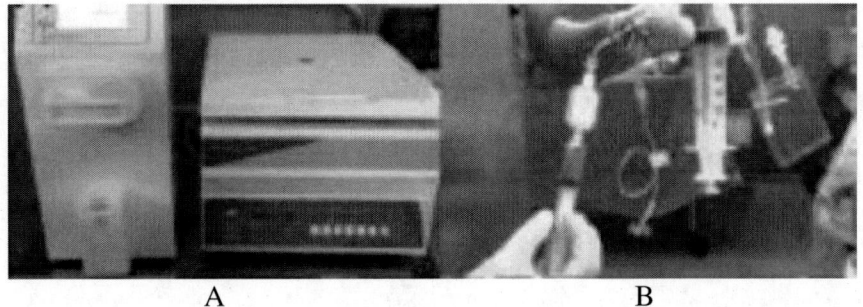

Figure 2. Platelet rich plasma preparation with C-Punt (A) Centrifuge and light selector. (B) C-punt device (Gentile 2017).

Then, autologous PRP, not activated obtained after centrifugation (9 ml), was switched with 10-ml tubes containing Ca2+.

Autologous PRP, not activated, obtained by the C-Punt procedure after centrifugation (20ml), was inserted in a light selector device. At the end of the procedure, 9ml of PRP was harvested.

In another study published in 2017 (Gentile 2017), the author compared his own experience using autologous Not-Activated PRP (A-PRP) obtained by C-Punt system with the use of Activated-PRP (AA-PRP) produced using a Regen Blood Cell Therapy tubes and the Arthrex Angel System.

Regen Blood Cell Therapy (BCT) tubes were used to prepare A-PRP (15mL, 5mL per BCT tube) from whole blood (24mL) taken from a peripheral vein using sodium citrate as an anticoagulant.

The top 2mL of A-PRP from each tube was then discarded, giving 9mL of A-PRP with a five-fold increase in platelet concentration over whole blood.

Similarly, the Arthrex Angel system was used to prepare A-PRP (3mL) from 120mL of whole blood when the instrument hematocrit level was set to 2%.

The A-PRP was then combined with 5 mL of platelet poor plasma to produce 8mL of A-PRP with a five-fold increase in platelet concentration over whole blood. A-PRP collected from both systems was then activated through the addition of 10% (v/v) calcium gluconate, which was immediately injected into the treatment zone.

More recently (Gentile 2019) the author prepared PRP from autologous blood (17.7mL) using the i-Stem Kit PRP Preparation System (i-Stem, Biostems, Co., LTD., Seoul, South Korea 138 - 843, Medical Device, CE and Food and Drug Administration (FDA)) (Figure 3) under the approval of the transfusional service. Sodium citrate (ACD) as an anticoagulant, was added (2.2mL).

After the first spin (centrifugation at 3000rpm for 6 min) the author removed the Platelet-Poor Plasma PPP portion (1mL) and RBC (Red blood cells) (2mL) and re-centrifuged for the second time (3000rpm for 3min) and at the end of the procedure, 15mL of A-PRP was obtained.

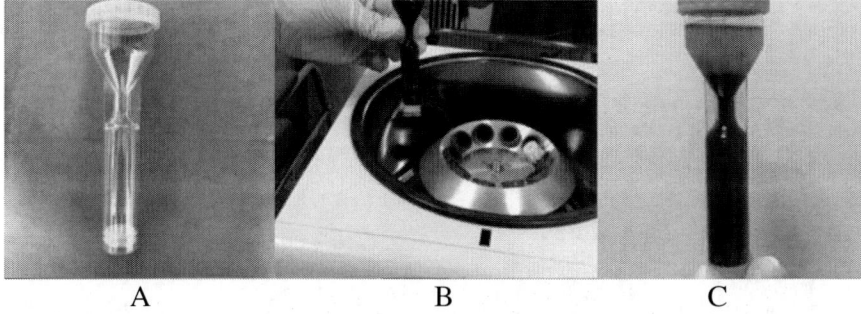

Figure 3. Platelet rich plasma preparation with the i-Stem Kit PRP Preparation (A) kit i-Stem; (B) Centrifuge; (C) i-stem device after the centrifugation (Gentile 2019).

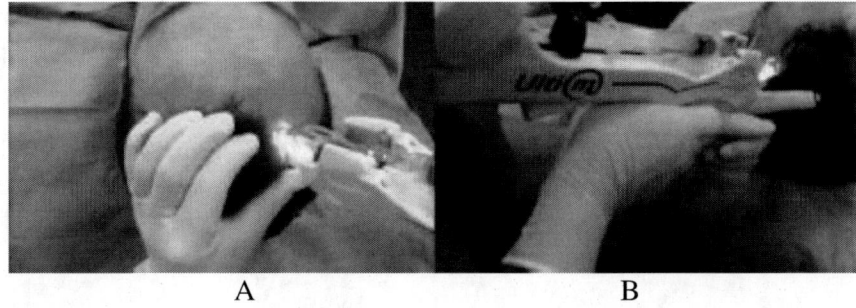

Figure 4. Platelet rich plasma injection with the mesotherapy gun. (A) Interfollicular PRP injections (0.2 mL/cm2) by Ultim-Gun (anti-Aging Medical System); (B) equipment with a 30 gauge and 10mL luer look syringe with PRP (Gentile 2017).

Platelet Rich Plasma Injections

As published (Gentile 2017) the scalp must be divided into six different anatomical areas (left frontal area, right frontal area, left parietal area, right parietal area, left vertex area and right vertex area); anesthesia (local or potentially fundamental) it is not necessary. The PRP suspension inter-follicular infusions (0.2mL/cm^2) must be injected to targeted area (TA) at 5mm depth utilizing a mesotherapy medical device outfitted with a 10mL syringe luer-lock with needle 30-gauge (Figure 4), in three sessions spaced 30 days apart.

Clinical Assessment of Hair Growth

Assessment of hair growth (HG) may be evaluated in different weeks (Ws) after the treatment, that could be summarized in four phases: T0, before the first infusion, T1 - 3 Ws, T2 - 9 Ws, T3 - 16 Ws, T4 - 23 Ws, T5 - 58 Ws after the last treatment.

The impacts of PRP interfollicular injection on HG must be evaluated using photography (same position, same contrast, same light), the physician's and patient's global evaluation scale, and standardized phototrichograms. In all parteciants, TA has been marked with a semi-permanent tattoo for the subsequent trichogram.

Phototrichogra were performed in all TA using Fotofinder videoepiluminescence systems in combination with the Trichoscan digital image analysis. TrichoScan evaluate hairs per $0.65cm^2$ described as hair count (HC), hairs per cm^2 described as hair density (HD), hair thickness (HT), anagen-to-telogen ratio, and vellus hair-to-terminal hair ratio. All hairs with a thickness > 40 μm are categorized as terminal hairs while those with lesser diameter are categorized as vellus hairs.

RESULTS

Clinical and Trichoscopic Results

Hair regrowth in a clinical evaluation demonstrated a positive reaction to treatment with A-PRP in patients showing significative improvements in hair density and hair count in the treated zone over the control zone (treated with the placebo). Differences between the 12-week follow-up hair counts and the baseline hair counts were observed. These hair growth parameters were higher in the A-PRP treatment group than in the AA-PRP treatment populace, as reported in past data published by Gentile et al. (Gentile 2018). Specifically, three-month hair density estimations for patients treated with A-PRP and AA-PRP were 65 ± 5 and 28 ± 4 hairs/cm^2, respectively.

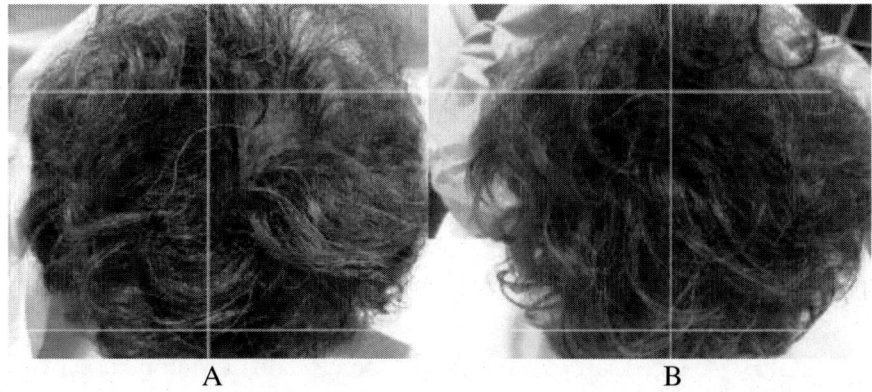

Figure 5. Non-smoker 34-year-old female affected by AGA classified in stage 2 according to Norwood-Hamilton scale. (a) Pre-operative image at T0 with thinning localized to the frontal and parietal areas; (b) Post-perative image 12 weeks later the last treatment); with increase of HD in right parietal area treated with (A-PRP) versus left parietal area treated with placebo (Gentile 2019).

The outcomes established a $31 \pm 2\%$ improvement in hair density when the A-PRP treatment was performed versus a $19 \pm 3\%$ improvement in hair density when the AA-PRP treatment was performed, with a significant difference in hair growth ($p = 0.0029$). The increase in the hair growth parameters for A-PRP over AA PRP may mirror the proficiency of in vivo thrombin in activating platelets and the body to distribute the contents of the activated platelets compared to in vitro calcium activation and infusion.

BIOMOLECULAR PATHWAY ANALYSIS

Biomolecular Pathway Analysis of Growth Factors Released by Platelet Rich Plasma

- EGF: Improves migration and growth of follicle ORS cells by the activation of Wnt/β-catenin signaling;
- TGF-β: Stimulates the signaling pathways that regulate hair cycle;

- IGF-1: Improves survival, migration, and proliferation of hair follicle cells;
- b-FGF: Improves the development of hairs' follicles;
- IL-6: Involved in WIHN through STAT3 activation;
- VEGF: Improves peri-follicular angiogenesis;
- PDGF and PDGFR-β/-α64: Up-regulate the genes involved in hair follicle differentiation. Induction and regulation of anagen. PDGF and its receptors are essential for follicular development;
- IGFBP-1 to -6: Regulates IGF-1 effects and its interaction with extracellular matrix proteins at the hair follicle level;
- BMP: Maintains DPC phenotype (crucial for stimulation of hair follicle stem cell);
- BMPR1a: Maintains the proper identity of DPCs (essential for specific DPC function);
- M-CSF: Involved in wound-induced hair re-growth;
- M-CSFR: Involved in wound-induced hair re-growth;
- Wnt3a: Involved in hair follicle development throug β-catenin signaling;
- PGE2: Stimulates anagen in hair follicles;
- PGF2α: and analogs improve the transition from telogen to anagen;
- BIO (GSK-3 inhibitor);
- PGE2 or inhibition of PGD2 or PGD2 receptor D2/ GPR4477: Improve follicle regeneration;

Talavera-Adame et al. (Talavera-Adame 2017), revealed in a recent study the bio-molecular pathway involved in a cellular treatment. Specifically, it has been additionally demonstrated that Wnt/β-catenin signaling is fundamental for the growth and upkeep of Dermal Papilla cells (DPCs). The increment of Wnt signaling in DPCs evidently is one of the principal factors that enhance hair re-growth.

In particular, in a study published by Pirastu N. et al. (Pirastu 2017), androgen receptor signaling, is implicated by seven genes at six loci. Three main groups were found: genes linked to Wnt signaling (RSPO2; LGR4; WNT10A; WNT3; DKK2; SOX13; TWIST2; TWIST1; IQGAP1; and PRKD1), genes involved in apoptosis (DFFA; BCL2; IRF4; TOP1; and MAPT) and a third more heterogeneous group including the androgen's receptor and TGF-β pathways (RUNX3; RUNX2; ALPL; PTHLH; RUNX1; AR; SRD5A2; PDGFA; PAX3; and FGF5). Although many different pathways have been implicated in the development of AGA, their results suggest that in addition to the androgen receptor pathway, for which they confirm a prominent function, the Wnt and apoptosis pathways play a fundamental role.

AGA is characterized by a shorter growth (anagen), which has been associated with increased apoptosis of the hair follicle cells. This result suggests the anagen phase becomes shorter because of differences in the genes regulating apoptosis.

The Wnt pathway has been implicated in the transition from the telogen (resting) to the anagen (growth), and also in the determination of the fate of the stem cells in the hair bulge, which are both dysregulated in balding tissue. Finally, baldness risk loci in the WNT ligand biogenesis and trafficking and Class B/2 (Secretin family receptors) pathways were also associated with height, despite none of the individual loci in these pathways being significant: this suggests a "pathway-wide" effect. Therefore, baldness shows pathway-specific genetic correlations, which provide a potential biological basis to observed epidemiological correlations.

Pathway-specific genetic correlations hold promise in disentangling the shared biological pathways underpinning complex diseases (Pirastu 2017).

CONCLUSION

The information reported in this chapter obviously highlights the constructive effects of Platelet rich plasma interfollicular injection in patients affected by AGA without major side effects.

REFERENCES

Gentile, P., Scioli, M. G., Bielli, A., De Angelis, B., De Sio, C., De Fazio, D., Ceccarelli, G., Trivisonno, A., Orlandi, A., Cervelli, V., Garcovich, S. (2019). Platelet-Rich Plasma and Micrografts Enriched with Autologous Human Follicle Mesenchymal Stem Cells Improve Hair Re-Growth in Androgenetic Alopecia. Biomolecular Pathway Analysis and Clinical Evaluation. *Biomedicines,* 8, 7, 2.

Gentile, P., Garcovich, S. (2019). Advances in Regenerative Stem Cell Therapy in Androgenic Alopecia and Hair Loss: Wnt pathway, Growth-Factor, and Mesenchymal Stem Cell Signaling Impact Analysis on Cell Growth and Hair Follicle Development. *Cells,* 16, 8, 5.

Gentile, P., Garcovich, S., Scioli, M. G., Bielli, A., Orlandi, A., Cervelli, V. (2018). Mechanical and Controlled PRP Injections in Patients Affected by Androgenetic Alopecia. *J. Vis. Exp.,* 27, 131.

Gentile, P., Cole, J. P., Cole, M. A., Garcovich, S., Bielli, A., Scioli, M. G., Orlandi, A., Insalaco, C., Cervelli, V. (2017). Evaluation of Not-Activated and Activated PRP in Hair Loss Treatment: Role of Growth Factor and Cytokine Concentrations Obtained by Different Collection Systems. *Int. J. Mol. Sci.,* 14, 18, 2.

Gentile, P., Garcovich, S., Bielli, A., Scioli, M. G., Orlandi, A., Cervelli, V. (2015). The Effect of Platelet-Rich Plasma in Hair Regrowth: A Randomized Placebo-Controlled Trial. *Stem Cells Transl. Med.,* 4, 11, 1317 - 23.

Gkini, M. A., Kouskoukis, A. E., Tripsianis, G. (2014). Study of platelet-rich plasma injections in the treatment of androgenetic alopecia through an one-year period. *J. Cutan. Aesthet. Surg.,* 7, 213 - 219.

Khatu, S. S., More, Y. E., Gokhale, N. R. (2014). Platelet-rich plasma in androgenic alopecia: myth or an effective tool. *J. Cutan. Aesthet. Surg.,* 7, 107 - 110.

Li, Z. J., Choi, H. I., Choi, D. K. (2012). Autologous platelet-rich plasma: A potential therapeutic tool for promoting hair growth. *Dermatol. Surg.,* 38, 1040 - 1046.

Pirastu, N., Joshi, P. K., de Vries, P. S., Cornelis, M. C., McKeigue, P. M., Keum, N. Franceschini, N., Colombo, M., Giovannucci, E. L., Spiliopoulou, A. et al. (2017). GWAS for male-pattern baldness identifies 71 susceptibility loci explaining 38% of the risk. *Nat. Commun.,* 8, 1584.

Talavera-Adame, D., Newman, D., Newman, N. (2017). Conventional and novel stem cell based therapies for androgenic alopecia. *Stem Cells Cloning,* 10, 11 - 19.

Trink, A., Sorbellini, E., Bezzola, P. et al. (2013). A randomized, double-blind, placebo- and activecontrolled, half-head study to evaluate the effects of platelet-rich plasma on alopecia areata. *Br. J. Dermatol.,* 169, 690 - 694.

Uebel, C. O., da Silva, J. B., Cantarelli, D., Martins, P. (2006). The role of platelet plasma growth factors in male pattern baldness surgery. *Plast. Reconstr. Surg.,* 118, 1458 - 1466.

In: Alopecia
Editor: Pietro Gentile
ISBN: 978-1-53617-008-5
© 2020 Nova Science Publishers, Inc.

Chapter 8

THREE - CO - FAT

Angelo Trivisonno[1,], Giovanni Trivisonno[2]
and Filippo Calcagni[1]*
[1]Private Practice Clinica Assunzione di Maria Santissima,
Rome, Italy
[2]Campus Biomedico University, Rome, Italy

ABSTRACT

In the last decades the adipose tissue has acquired an important role in the regenerative field, including hair re-growth. It is important to choose the best tissue for this purpose and the best procedure. The adipose tissue is not uniform. There are differences in relation to the sites of the body, and even to different depth. The choose of the sites and the depth, morever of the types of cannulas and the products of the fat employed, and the correct plane to inject is considered in this chapter.

Keywords: ADSC, SVF cells, adipose tissue, superficial adipose tissue, regenerative medicine, hair regrowth

---

* Corresponding Author's Email: dott.a.trivisonno@gmail.com.

INTRODUCTION

In particular several recent studies have considered that the adipocyte lineage in the superficial fat forms a niche influencing the epithelial stem cells behavior. This superficial fat closed to deep dermis is considered Dermal White Adipose Tissue (DWAT), to distinguish it from the deeper Subcutaneous White Adipose Tissue (SWAT) (Driskell 2014; Trivisonno 2017). In particular the fat around the hair follicles interacts with them to influence hair growth. In fact patients with dystrophy, or other diseases such as obesity, or anorexia, show hair follicles growth defects (Fukumoto 2009). Normally the turnover of the adipose tissue is slow, while in the DWAT the turnover is faster and the adipogenesis move parallelly to hair follicles growth. During Anagen the fat thickness is double, but does not due to an hypertrophy, but a real proliferation of adipocytes precursors. So there is a real adipogenesis (Festa 2011).

At nowadays some pathways of this communication are known as the Shh and the Wnt pathway signaling, that stimulate hair follicle stem cells to cycle. The Bone Morphogenic Protein (BMP) released in this microenvironment produces inhibition of the hair follicles activity and inhibits the Wnt pathway signaling (Jahoda 2011). The PDGFA conversely stimulates hair growth.

Considering all this, it is evident that the fat around the follicles is the best choice for hair regeneration purpose. The aim of this chapter was report the preliminar experience in the use of different kinds of fat as macrofat, microfat and nanofat gel called THREE – CO – FAT.

METHODS

Procedure and Patients

So, the first author of this chapter, Trivisonno, designed a microcannula with small holes arranged on a single raw, that allows to harvest selectively the fat upwards in contact with deep dermis. In this way it was possible to harvest this fat around the follicles, for example in pubis area, without skin damages (Trivisonno 2014).

After decantation it was possible to remove the oil on the top and the fluid in the bottom of the syringe, to keep only the middle part, with alive tissue.

This superficial fat harvesting was injected by 1 cc syringes, through a 1,2mm microcannula, in the superficial plane of the scalp, in the area where it was ncessary stimulate the follicles, to improve the quality of the scalp, and in the area where we need obtain regenerative results, including angiogenesis.

The authors considered to use 3 types of fat products: macrofat, microfat and nanofat gel, to inject in 3 different planes. They called this procedure "THREE – CO -FAT".

The procedure consists in the harvesting around 40 - 50 cc of macrofat by macrocannula with holes of almost 2mm of diameter, in the lateral thigh, or flank and harvesting around 15-20 cc of microfat by Trivisonno microcannula, in the superficial layer of fat, in area with hairs, like pubis, or abdomen.

20 cc of macrofat were processed by transfer and nanotransfer, or lipocube device, to obtain nanofat. Then the nanofat was centrifuged to 3000 RPM for 3 minutes.

So it was possible to separate 3 layers: the yellow oil on the top, the red liquid on the bottom of the syringe, and in the middle a smaller white layer of SVF cells and Extracellular Matrix. This white layer represent 1/10 of the total volume.

Then, it was used a suspension of 20-30 cc of macrofat to inject by 1,5 mm microcannula in deep plane of the scalp to restore the thinner subcutaneous layer. This created a soft and more vascularized environment for the dermal papillae. After the microfat harvested in superficial layer of fat, was injected by 1,2mm microcannula in superficial plane of the scalp. At last the nanogel was injected by 27 Gauge needle into the dermis of the scalp. 15 patients were treated with this procedure (Figures 1, 2) and they were evaluated by trichogram (Figures 3, 4) with good results.

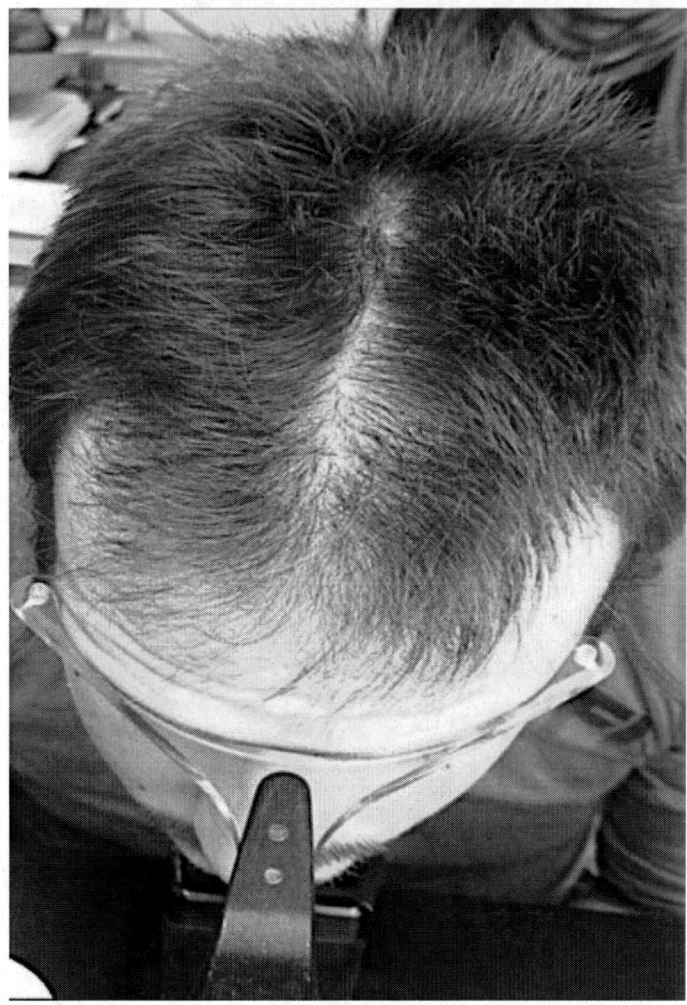

Figure 1. Pre operative view.

RESULTS

Clinical and Trichoscopic Results

In this chapter the results obtained displayed an improvement in the mean hair count after 24 weeks (24 weeks vs. 0 weeks) of 13.0 hairs in the treated area (Figure 4) compared with baseline (Figure 3). Accordingly, a mean increase in total hair density of 17.6 hairs per cm^2 (Figure 4) compared with baseline (Figure 3) was observed at the same time.

Following 12 months, 6 patients detailed dynamic hair loss. Those six patients were re-treated.

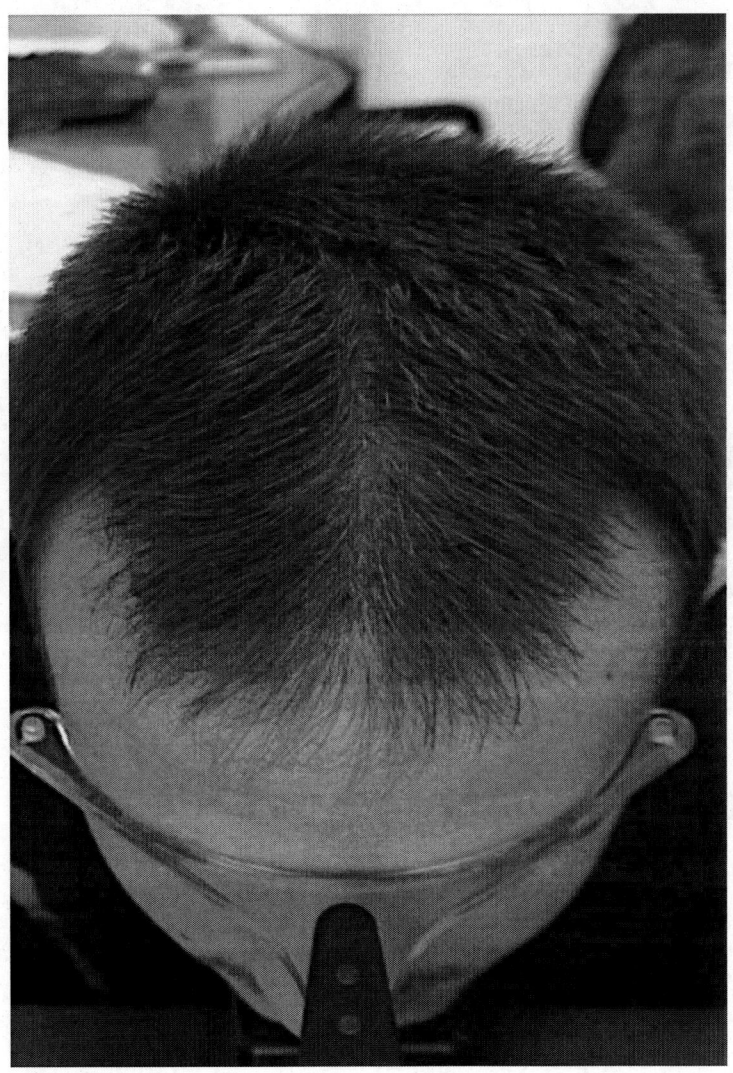

Figure 2. Postoperative view 1 year.

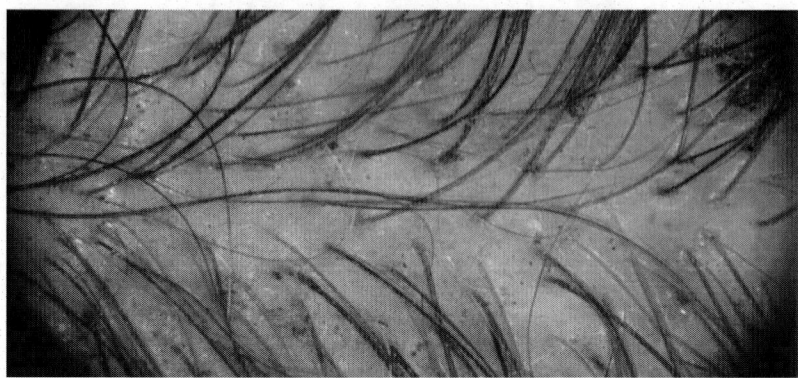

Figure 3. Pre operative trichogram.

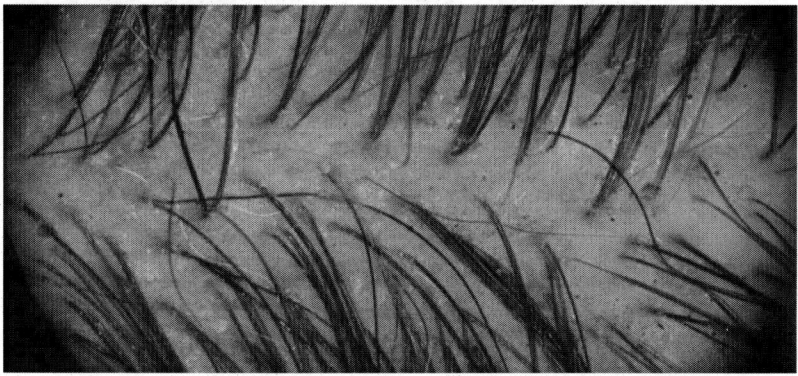

Figure 4. Post operative trichogram.

REFERENCES

Driskell, R. R., Jahoda, C. A., Chuong, C. M., Watt, F. M., Horsley, V. (2014). Defining dermal adipose tissue. *Exp. Dermatol.*, 23, 9, 629 - 31.

Festa, E., Fretz, J., Berry, R., Schmidt, B., Rodeheffer, M., Horowitz, M., Horsley, V. (2011). Adipocyte lineage cells contribute to the skin stem cell niche to drive hair cycling. *Cell*, 2,146,5,761 - 71.

Fukumoto, D., Kubo, Y., Saito, M., Arase, S. (2009). Centrifugal lipodystrophy of the scalp presenting with an arch-form alopecia: a 10-year follow-up observation. *J. Dermatol.*, 36,9,499 - 503.

Jahoda, C. A., Christiano, A. M. (2011). Niche crosstalk: intercellular signals at the hair follicle. *Cell*, 2,146,5,678 - 81.

Trivisonno, A., Rossi, A., Monti, M., Di Nunno, D., Desouches, C., Cannistra, C., Toietta, G. (2017). Facial skin rejuvenation by autologous dermal microfat transfer in photoaged patients: Clinical evaluation and skin surface digital profilometry analysis. *J. Plast. Reconstr. Aesthet. Surg.,* 70, 8, 1118 - 1128.

Trivisonno, A., Di Rocco, G., Cannistra, C., Finocchi, V., Torres Farr, S., Monti, M., Toietta, G. (2014). Harvest of superficial layers of fat with a microcannula and isolation of adipose tissue-derived stromal and vascular cells. *Aesthet. Surg. J.,* 1,34,4,601 - 13.

In: Alopecia
Editor: Pietro Gentile

ISBN: 978-1-53617-008-5
© 2020 Nova Science Publishers, Inc.

Chapter 9

FDA AND EUROPEAN RULES REGARDING USE OF ADIPOSE DERIVED-STROMAL VASCULAR CELLS (AD-SVFS) AND HUMAN FOLLICLE MESENCHYMAL STEM CELLS (HF-MSCS) IN HAIR RE-GROWTH

Laura Dionisi[*]

Biotechnology Rules and Recommendations, Rome, Italy

ABSTRACT

Treatments for hair re-growth based on new biotechnologies as adipose derived-stromal vascular fraction cells (AD-SVFs) and human follicle mesenchymal stem cells (HF-MSCs) must be established performing detailed anamnesis, therapeutic history (i.e., screening for drugs linked to hair loss), clinical examination, blood test, urinalysis, and trichoscopic highlights evaluating specific exclusion and inclusion

---

[*] Corresponding Author's Email: studio@avvocatolauradionisi.it.

criteria. In each case, these strategies must be used respecting the FDA and European rules.

INTRODUCTION

The U. S. Food and Drug Administration (FDA) and the European Medicines Agency (EMA) consider grown-up cell products as biological products that are isolated into two classes: minimally manipulated biological products and manipulated biological products. Regulation number 1394/2007 of the European Parliament for cutting-edge treatments defines "bioprocess engineering products," which excludes products that contain or are made solely of cells and non-vital human or animal tissues that do not have pharmacological, immunologic, or metabolic activity. Included amongst the advanced therapy pharmaceutical products are ones used for gene and somatic cell treatment (Directive 2001/83/European Parliament, Annex I). The aim of the present chapter is to describe the rules must be respected in cells-based therapy reported by FDA and EMA.

This chapter would also provide a concise review of recent advances in this field.

MINIMAL AND EXTENSIVE MANIPULATION

Cells and tissues are to be viewed as results of the bioprocess engineering products in the event that they experience "extensive manipulation." This rule contrasts between extensive and minimal manipulation. Manipulations that are not considered as bioprocess engineering include the following: cutting, granulating, forming, purification, centrifugation, absorbing anti-toxins or antimicrobial arrangements, cleansing, lighting, partition, fixation or decontamination, filtration, lyophilization, solidifying cryopreservation, and nitrification.

The definition of medicines for advanced therapy excludes non-repetitive preparations completed under the supervision of a doctor running an individual remedy for a product explicitly intended for that specific patient, without obviously disregarding the important standards that identify with quality and security.

Further to the execution of Article 17 of Regulation (EC) No 1394/2007 (the Advanced Therapy Medicinal Products (ATMPs) Regulation), applicants are required to approach the Committee for Advanced Therapies (CAT) with a logical proposal for the arrangement of ATMPs. The committee is in charge of surveying the quality, well-being, and viability of cutting-edge treatment medications, including medications delegated as quality treatment, substantial cell treatment, or tissue-built products. CAT is supported by the ATMP regulation, which empowers the EMA in a joint effort with the European Commission to decide if a given product meets the logical criteria that characterize ATMPs. The ATMP grouping technique was introduced with the goal of addressing inquiries into situations where the arrangement of a product dependent on genes, cells, or tissues is not clear. The CAT issues logical proposals to determine if the product falls within the definition of an ATMP in the European Union. The ATMP Regulation and Directive 2001/83/EC Annex I Part IV provide exact legal definitions of ATMPs.

The ATMP characterization depends on an assessment of whether a given product satisfies one of the characteristics of gene therapy medicinal products (GTMP), somatic cell therapy medicinal products (sCTMPs), or tissue engineered products (TEPs), and whether that product satisfies the definition of a consolidated ATMP. It is additionally recognized that, because of the complex nature of these restorative products, the constrained information bundle at the beginning period of the product improvement, as well as the rapid growth of science and innovation, may result in inquiries off the fringe.

EMA/CAT Recommendations on Minimal Manipulation

According to the reflection paper on the portrayal of front-line treatment therapeutic products, EMA/CAT/600280/2010 Rev 1, June 20, 2014, by the Committee for Advanced Therapies (CAT), Line 10, "a similar basic capacity for a cell populace implies that the cells, when expelled from their unique condition in the human body are used to maintain the original capacity in a similar anatomical or histological condition." The authors presumed autologous application in a one-stage medical procedure, minimal manipulation, omofunctional use "used for an indistinguishable fundamental capacity in the beneficiary as in the donor," and manipulation with devices in aseptic conditions would be conditions that do not require good manufacturing practice (GMP) rules for preparation, good clinical practices (GCP) for the clinical application, or ethical committee underwriting.

Italian Rules Regarding Platelet-Rich Plasma Use

Platelet-rich plasma (PRP) preparation must be performed in Italy respecting the Decree of the Blood, November 2, 2015, dispositions related to quality, and safety parameters for blood and emocomponents.

References

Article 17 of Regulation (EC) No 1394/2007 (the Advanced Therapy Medicinal Products (ATMPs) Regulation).
Directive 2001/83/European Parliament, Annex I.
Reflection paper EMA/CAT/600280/2010 Rev. 1, June 20, 2014, by the Committee for Advanced Therapies (CAT).

Regulation number 1394/2007 of the European Parliament for cutting-edge treatments.

The ATMP Regulation and Directive 2001/83/EC Annex I Part IV.

Editor's Contact Information

Pietro Gentile, MD, PhD
Regenerative Plastic Surgeon,
Researcher of Plastic and Reconstructive Surgery
Via Courmayeur, Rome, Italy
Email: pietrogentile2004@libero.it

INDEX

A

acid, 39, 71, 78, 90, 107
adipocyte, 83, 93, 94, 108, 109, 111, 124, 148
adipose, 81, 82, 86, 91, 92, 93, 94, 97, 98, 99, 101, 102, 104, 105, 106, 107, 109, 110, 111, 129, 147, 148, 152, 153, 155
adipose mesenchymal stem cells, 82, 91, 98
adipose tissue, 92, 94, 98, 102, 106, 107, 109, 110, 129, 147, 148, 152, 153
adipose-derived stem cells (ADSC), 92, 93, 94, 99, 101, 102, 104, 147
adolescents, 4, 42, 50, 56
adults, 31, 37, 40, 41, 42, 43
adverse effects, 40, 41, 42, 45
adverse event, 42, 44
age, 2, 3, 4, 6, 8, 9, 21, 22, 31, 33, 82
alexithymia, 1, 2, 4, 5, 7, 8, 9, 12, 13, 14, 15, 16, 17, 18, 19, 20
alopecia, , 2, 3, 4, 5, 6, 7, 8, 9, 11, 12, 13, 14, 15, 16, 17, 18, 19, 20, 21, 22, 27, 28, 29, 30, 31, 32, 33, 34, 35, 36, 37, 39, 40, 41, 42, 43, 44, 45, 46, 47, 48, 49, 50, 51, 52, 53, 54, 55, 56, 57, 58, 59, 63, 66, 68, 69, 70, 72, 73, 74, 75, 76, 77, 78, 79, 82, 83, 85, 99, 101, 102, 103, 113, 114, 115, 119, 129, 130, 131, 132, 135, 144, 145, 152
alopecia areata, 1, 2, 3, 10, 12, 15, 17, 18, 19, 29, 30, 31, 32, 33, 34, 35, 36, 37, 39, 40, 41, 42, 43, 44, 45, 46, 47, 48, 49, 50, 51, 52, 53, 54, 55, 56, 57, 58, 59, 63, 66, 70, 72, 76, 77, 78, 79, 82, 83, 99, 119, 132, 145
alternative treatments, 81, 86
amnion, 89, 109
amniotic fluid, 89, 90, 91, 99, 107, 111
amniotic mesenchymal stem cells, 82, 98
anchorage, 68, 69
androgen, 27, 67, 85, 104, 142
androgenic alopecia, 33, 130, 144, 145
angiogenesis, 88, 94, 99, 119, 132, 136, 142, 149
anticoagulant, 137, 138
anxiety, 1, 2, 3, 4, 6, 8, 9, 11, 12, 14, 15, 16, 30, 35, 48, 55, 82
apoptosis, 25, 45, 72, 97, 99, 108, 143
aseptic, 89, 134, 158
assessment, 6, 18, 30, 157
asymptomatic, 32, 33
atopic dermatitis, 30, 48, 86
atopy, 35, 49
atrophy, 37, 38

autoimmune disease, 3, 35, 74
autoimmune diseases, 35

B

base, 82, 87
basement membrane, 68, 69, 74
beneficial effect, 66, 93, 110
benefits, 30, 36, 49
biological fluids, 96, 109
biopsy, 65, 116, 117, 121
biotechnology, 26, 102
blood, 22, 23, 65, 73, 74, 86, 89, 116, 133, 136, 137, 138, 155, 158
blood supply, 73, 74
bone, 83, 92, 96, 97, 99, 107, 108, 111, 121
bone marrow, 92, 96, 97, 99, 107, 108, 111, 121
brain, 62, 65, 78

C

Ca^{2+}, 137, 138
calcium, 87, 88, 135, 137, 138, 141
capillary, 83, 94
carbohydrates, 66, 67, 90
cell culture, 89, 96, 99, 105, 109
cell line, 88, 90, 91, 99, 101
cell lines, 88, 91, 99, 101
cell signaling, 95, 102
cell surface, 84, 92
chemokines, 86, 135
childhood, 30, 49, 52
children, 4, 31, 32, 37, 40, 42, 43, 50, 51, 53, 54, 56, 78
clinical application, 81, 87, 88, 96, 134, 158
clinical examination, 22, 23, 64, 66, 116, 133, 155
clinical trials, 86, 98
closure, 90, 101
collaboration, 123

collagen, 92, 97, 119, 136
commercial, 26, 87, 89, 96, 98, 134
composition, 92, 98
connective tissue, 66, 120
control group, 2, 3, 5, 8, 11, 12, 44
controlled studies, 128
correlation, 8, 9, 12, 79
correlations, 26, 143
corticosteroid therapy, 38, 40, 58
corticosteroids, 30, 36, 37, 38, 40, 43, 44, 49
cosmetic, 45, 48
cryopreservation, 89, 92, 106, 133, 156
cues, 84, 88, 136
cultivation, 106
culture, 46, 89, 92, 94, 97, 98, 120, 121, 122, 123
culture conditions, 94, 98, 122
culture media, 89
cycles, 38, 100, 122
cycling, 93, 97, 102, 128, 135, 152
cyclosporine, 41, 53, 59
cytokines, 86, 87, 89, 90, 93, 104

D

deficiencies, 62, 66, 70, 82
degradation, 84, 95
deposition, 91, 92, 104
depression, 1, 2, 3, 4, 5, 6, 8, 9, 11, 12, 14, 15, 16, 18, 30, 35, 48, 55, 67, 82, 107
depth, 117, 118, 139, 147
dermatitis, 40, 44, 48, 63
dermatology, 5, 57, 61, 62, 63, 73
dermis, 83, 91, 105, 148, 149
diabetes, 27, 36, 74, 99, 103
diet, 66, 70, 71, 72, 74, 79
dieting, 64, 73
diseases, 2, 26, 43, 65, 97, 143, 148
disorder, 3, 21, 22, 35, 66, 67, 82
distribution, 9, 12, 13, 33, 58

diversity, 109
dosage, 37, 91
draft, 134
drugs, 23, 40, 155

E

ECM, 114, 124
emotion, 4, 48
engineering, 113, 156
environment, 72, 74, 79, 149
epidemiologic, 35
epidermis, 105, 116, 122, 130
epithelial cells, 97, 99, 123
epithelium, 85, 93, 104
ESCs, 114, 121, 122, 123
ester, 39, 71
etiology, 35, 82
European Parliament, 114, 134, 156, 158, 159
evidence, 30, 37, 44, 65, 89, 131, 136
exclusion, 96, 155
execution, 116, 157
exosomes, 81, 82, 86, 95, 96, 97, 98, 100, 103, 104, 105, 108, 109, 111
exposure, 39, 45, 94
extracellular matrix, 104, 124, 142
extraction, 73, 77

F

families, 30, 95
family history, 30, 34, 49
fat, 74, 103, 105, 111, 116, 124, 147, 148, 149, 153
FDA, 21, 22, 23, 24, 67, 92, 132, 138, 155, 156
feelings, 2, 3, 4, 7, 48
ferritin, 67, 75
fibroblast growth factor, 85, 88, 109, 133, 135

fibroblast proliferation, 91, 97
fibroblasts, 85, 90, 93, 136
fibrosis, 90, 97, 108
fluid, 89, 91, 110, 149
follicle, 22, 31, 73, 82, 83, 84, 85, 88, 91, 93, 102, 106, 107, 114, 115, 122, 123, 129, 130, 141, 142, 155
follicles, 22, 30, 31, 32, 61, 62, 68, 69, 71, 82, 91, 93, 111, 115, 132, 135, 136, 142, 148, 149
Food and Drug Administration, 21, 22, 132, 138, 156
formation, 85, 95, 129, 130
fragments, 116, 117, 121

G

gel, 148, 149
generalized anxiety disorder, 3, 48
genes, 25, 30, 35, 52, 84, 104, 142, 143, 157
genetic information, 106
glucocorticoids, 38, 40, 41, 70
granules, 24, 87, 88, 98, 132, 135
growth, 3, 25, 30, 31, 37, 39, 40, 41, 44, 52, 57, 62, 64, 67, 68, 69, 71, 74, 78, 82, 83, 85, 86, 87, 88, 89, 90, 91, 93, 94, 97, 98, 99, 100, 101, 102, 103, 104, 105, 106, 107, 109, 110, 113, 115, 118, 119, 122, 124, 129, 130, 131, 132, 133, 135, 136, 140, 141, 142, 143, 144, 145, 147, 148, 155, 157
growth factor, 44, 68, 69, 74, 86, 87, 88, 89, 90, 93, 98, 99, 101, 102, 105, 106, 119, 130, 132, 135, 145

H

hair follicle, 22, 23, 25, 30, 31, 36, 49, 66, 68, 69, 71, 72, 73, 78, 82, 83, 85, 87, 88, 91, 93, 94, 97, 99, 100, 102, 104, 106,

107, 108, 110, 111, 115, 121, 128, 129, 130, 136, 142, 143, 148, 153
hair loss, 3, 6, 21, 22, 23, 24, 27, 28, 30, 31, 32, 33, 36, 38, 40, 41, 42, 43, 45, 48, 49, 55, 62, 63, 64, 65, 66, 67, 68, 71, 73, 77, 78, 79, 81, 82, 83, 85, 86, 98, 99, 100, 101, 102, 109, 114, 115, 122, 124, 126, 127, 128, 129, 131, 132, 135, 151, 155
hair regrowth, 24, 28, 30, 38, 39, 40, 41, 42, 43, 45, 53, 55, 72, 88, 102, 140, 144, 147
hairless, 22, 115
halos, 66, 71
harvesting, 74, 116, 149
healing, 24, 68, 91
health, 46, 47, 48, 50, 57, 58, 65, 66, 82, 86
health care, 82, 86
height, 25, 143
herpes, 43, 63
herpes zoster, 43, 63
history, 6, 22, 32, 64, 66, 73, 116, 133, 155
hormone, 23, 61, 62, 65, 69
hormones, 35, 65, 90
Hospital Anxiety and Depression Scale (HADS), 2, 4, 6, 7, 8, 9, 16, 17
host, 63, 95
human, 78, 88, 89, 90, 94, 97, 99, 103, 104, 105, 106, 107, 108, 111, 115, 121, 122, 123, 129, 130, 136, 155, 156, 158
human body, 158
human skin, 107, 122, 130
hydrocortisone, 38, 53
hypothyroidism, 70, 74

I

identical twins, 30, 35
image, 25, 68, 119, 126, 127, 140, 141
image analysis, 25, 119, 140
immunomodulatory, 39, 89
immunotherapy, 30, 38, 39, 40, 53, 59
improvements, 24, 87, 94, 140

in vitro, 104, 108, 141
in vivo, 104, 122, 123, 141
induction, 45, 82, 94, 100, 122, 130
infection, 43, 92
inflammation, 30, 31, 35, 66, 92, 96, 107
inflammatory disease, 31, 49
inhibition, 42, 59, 71, 84, 85, 104, 142, 148
inhibitor, 23, 41, 42, 54, 59, 94, 115, 142
injections, 30, 36, 37, 45, 70, 87, 94, 97, 103, 114, 116, 119, 126, 127, 131, 132, 133, 139, 144
insulin, 88, 99, 132, 135
intervention, 36, 62, 75
iron, 23, 66, 67, 75, 82
irradiation, 98
isolation, 81, 96, 99, 102, 105, 120, 129, 153
issues, 67, 157
Italy, 21, 113, 131, 134, 147, 155, 158, 161

K

keratin, 94, 123
keratinocyte, 121
keratinocytes, 85, 88, 111, 114, 121, 123, 135, 136

L

lead, 30, 35, 36, 44, 73
leukocytes, 134, 137
lichen, 70, 79
lichen planus, 70, 79
lifetime, 3, 4, 31, 48
ligand, 25, 85, 143
light, 25, 39, 45, 67, 98, 110, 119, 137, 138, 140
lipids, 90, 95, 96
liver, 65, 97, 108
loci, 25, 28, 35, 36, 142, 143, 145
lymphocytes, 22, 30, 58, 115

lymphoma, 64

M

machinery, 95
major depression, 3
major depressive disorder, 4, 48
majority, 44, 122, 123
malignancy, 43, 45
management, 16, 36, 49, 53, 55, 78, 100
manipulation, 115, 120, 121, 134, 156, 158
marrow, 92, 97, 99
mast cells, 22, 31, 115
matrix, 83, 91, 98, 114, 132
matter, 96, 123
media, 89, 90, 91, 93, 94, 96, 97, 98, 99, 101, 109
medical, 4, 23, 28, 45, 48, 62, 73, 75, 92, 115, 117, 118, 121, 133, 135, 136, 139, 158
mental health, 47, 48, 107
mesenchymal stem cells, 82, 89, 91, 96, 98, 106, 107, 108, 111, 114, 121, 130, 155
meta-analysis, 30, 39, 41, 53, 55, 56
methylprednisolone, 53, 76
mice, 97, 105, 108, 110, 123
micronutrients, 64, 66
migration, 68, 90, 95, 97, 104, 111, 141, 142
miniaturization, 24, 115
modifications, 87, 137
molecules, 31, 88, 95, 124
mood disorder, 8, 12, 15
Moon, 45, 50, 104, 111
multipotent, 90, 106, 130

N

NaCl, 115, 116
negative effects, 48
neuroendocrine system, 79

nutrients, 64, 73, 90
nutrition, 23, 75
nutritional deficiencies, 62, 75

O

obesity, 103, 148
obsessive-compulsive disorder, 48
oligomers, 79
organ, 62, 65, 104
organs, 65, 90
outpatients, 7, 8, 9

P

pain, 47, 64, 90
parents, 36, 48, 49, 56
participants, 23
partition, 156
pathogenesis, 50, 57, 62, 75, 77, 129
pathology, 82
pathway, 25, 27, 42, 83, 85, 86, 95, 102, 105, 108, 123, 132, 142, 143, 144, 148
pathways, 25, 83, 85, 86, 88, 97, 104, 108, 143, 148
peptide, 70, 72, 75
peptides, 67, 90
personality, 3, 5
pilot study, 43, 50, 54, 77
placebo, 26, 27, 30, 37, 45, 50, 55, 56, 58, 102, 109, 116, 126, 127, 131, 133, 136, 140, 141, 145
plaque, 51, 58, 100
platelet rich plasma, 26, 61, 62, 68, 72, 73, 74, 75, 77, 79, 81, 82, 86, 100, 101, 131, 133, 134, 135, 136, 137, 139, 141, 143
platelets, 24, 87, 98, 132, 135, 141
population, 4, 14, 42, 48, 89, 91, 92, 93, 96, 130
positive correlation, 4, 5

preparation, 89, 98, 101, 114, 117, 118, 120, 132, 133, 134, 135, 137, 139, 158
progenitor cell, 92, 93, 115, 129
progenitor cells, 92, 93, 115, 129
prognosis, 35, 49
proliferation, 44, 88, 90, 94, 95, 97, 99, 109, 110, 111, 130, 133, 135, 136, 142, 148
prostaglandin, 44, 67
proteins, 24, 64, 66, 74, 84, 86, 88, 90, 95, 99, 136, 142
pruritus, 32, 48
psoriasis, 5, 30, 48, 51, 52, 58, 86
psychiatric disorder, 2, 3, 4, 5
psychiatric disorders, 2, 3, 5
psychological, 1, 2, 3, 5, 16, 17, 18, 30, 35, 47
psychopathology, 16
purification, 96, 100, 156

Q

quality of life, 1, 16, 26, 30, 34, 46, 50, 51, 52, 53, 54, 55, 56, 57, 58
questionnaire, 46, 47, 51

R

radiation, 30, 63
reactive oxygen, 66
receptor, 84, 85, 142
receptors, 25, 65, 84, 85, 142, 143
recommendations, iv, 62, 120
recovery, 92, 96
recurrence, 40, 41, 66, 72
regenerate, 123, 124
regeneration, 81, 88, 91, 93, 94, 97, 98, 102, 103, 104, 107, 108, 109, 122, 123, 128, 129, 142, 148
regenerative medicine, 24, 90, 92, 95, 98, 105, 131, 147
regression, 82, 83

regrowth, 24, 30, 33, 36, 37, 38, 39, 40, 41, 42, 43, 44, 45, 49, 53, 55, 72, 88, 91, 102, 140, 147
rejection, 92
relevance, 78, 91, 95
reliability, 6, 47
reparation, 135, 136
resistance, 35, 67
resolution, 65, 66
response, 5, 24, 37, 38, 39, 40, 41, 42, 44, 45, 65
rheumatoid arthritis, 36, 59, 86, 110, 111
risk, 4, 25, 28, 30, 31, 34, 35, 37, 43, 66, 86, 88, 89, 92, 95, 143, 145
risks, 36, 49, 91
root, 64, 82, 83, 88, 97, 99
rules, 115, 120, 133, 136, 156, 158

S

safety, 27, 58, 78, 86, 124, 131, 134, 158
science, 52, 157
secretion, 90, 95, 104
self-destruction, 65
self-esteem, 2, 3, 48, 82
sensations, 4, 7
sensitization, 39, 51
serum, 23, 27, 65, 70, 78, 89
serum ferritin, 23, 78
sex, 6, 9, 33
showing, 66, 132, 140
side effects, 24, 30, 37, 38, 40, 67, 81, 86, 91, 98, 127, 131, 143
signal transduction, 104
signaling pathway, 82, 83, 90, 94, 95, 97, 111, 123, 141
signalling, 105, 110
signals, 31, 62, 65, 68, 69, 72, 83, 122, 153
signs, 33, 42, 65
skin, 27, 30, 32, 37, 38, 39, 40, 46, 47, 48, 52, 56, 64, 65, 66, 70, 71, 72, 74, 76, 77,

78, 79, 83, 86, 93, 97, 99, 100, 102, 103, 105, 106, 119, 123, 128, 130, 149, 152, 153
smooth muscle, 92, 122
sodium, 137, 138
solution, 24, 26, 39, 44, 51, 69, 72, 76, 94, 115, 116, 117
somatic cell, 156, 157
spin, 87, 138
starvation, 64, 65
state, 64, 82, 83, 85, 87, 103
states, 65, 84, 86
stem cells, 25, 68, 69, 74, 75, 82, 84, 89, 90, 91, 92, 93, 94, 98, 99, 100, 101, 102, 104, 105, 106, 109, 110, 111, 114, 115, 121, 122, 128, 129, 130, 132, 143, 148
steroids, 56, 70
stimulation, 101, 142
stress, 35, 62, 64, 65, 73, 76
stromal cells, 90, 104, 106, 108, 124
structure, 90, 122, 123
Sun, 101, 107, 108, 111, 128, 130
superficial adipose tissue, 147
suppression, 31, 37, 38, 88, 94
survival, 69, 74, 97, 135, 142
susceptibility, 4, 28, 35, 145
SVF cells, 147, 149
symptoms, 3, 45, 46, 48, 55, 64
syndrome, 34, 63, 67
syphilis, 23, 33, 82, 89

T

T cell, 30, 31, 35, 36, 45, 64
T lymphocytes, 31, 59, 71
target, 84, 85, 96, 99
TAS-20, 2, 5, 7, 8, 9, 12, 16, 19
techniques, 5, 73, 89, 92, 96
testosterone, 23, 85
texture, 65, 70, 71, 72
TGF, 90, 132, 135, 141, 143

therapy, 22, 24, 25, 26, 27, 35, 37, 38, 40, 41, 43, 44, 45, 50, 52, 53, 55, 59, 61, 62, 66, 67, 68, 69, 70, 71, 72, 73, 74, 75, 76, 77, 78, 90, 92, 99, 100, 101, 102, 120, 124, 156, 157
thinning, 22, 66, 119, 124, 126, 127, 141
thrombin, 87, 88, 141
thyroid, 23, 65, 78, 82
tissue, 25, 64, 65, 74, 88, 89, 90, 91, 92, 94, 97, 98, 102, 106, 107, 109, 110, 114, 115, 116, 121, 122, 123, 128, 136, 143, 147, 148, 149, 152, 153, 157
tissue engineering, 106, 122, 128
totalis, 30, 32, 39, 41, 42, 43, 44, 45, 49, 53, 56, 57, 58, 71
trafficking, 25, 143
transcription, 85, 91, 97, 122
transcription factors, 85, 122
transforming growth factor, 132, 135
translocation, 84, 85, 97
transplant, 61, 62, 69, 72, 74, 75, 77, 79, 107
transplantation, 76, 99, 107, 129
trauma, 64, 73, 119
treatment, 2, 3, 5, 22, 23, 24, 25, 26, 27, 28, 30, 34, 36, 37, 38, 39, 40, 41, 42, 43, 45, 49, 50, 51, 52, 54, 55, 56, 57, 58, 59, 61, 62, 65, 67, 69, 73, 75, 76, 77, 78, 79, 81, 82, 87, 90, 91, 92, 93, 97, 98, 101, 102, 103, 114, 118, 125, 126, 127, 128, 130, 131, 132, 133, 134, 135, 138, 140, 141, 142, 144, 156, 157, 158
trial, 26, 38, 43, 44, 50, 53, 55, 69, 76, 79, 99, 102
triggers, 5, 31, 61, 62, 63, 65, 75
tumours, 64, 106

U

ultraviolet irradiation, 62, 65
uniform, 147

United States, 6, 92
universalis, 30, 32, 39, 41, 42, 43, 44, 45, 49, 50, 51, 53, 56, 57, 58, 71
urinalysis, 22, 116, 133, 155

V

valuation, 27, 144
vascular endothelial growth factor, 88, 132
vascular endothelial growth factor (VEGF), 88, 132
vascularization, 87, 136
VEGF, 74, 93, 94, 115, 135, 142
vein, 137, 138
video microscopy, 71
vitamin C, 94
vitamin D, 65, 66, 67, 75
vitamins, 66, 67, 74
vitiligo, 35, 40, 70

W

Wnt signaling, 85, 104, 124, 142, 143
World Health Organization, 46
worldwide, 102
wound healing, 86, 90, 94, 97, 99, 100, 105, 107, 111

Z

zinc, 66, 67, 70, 82

Related Nova Publications

NATURAL ANTI-AGING PLANTS AND DELAY OF SENESCENCE

EDITOR: Noboru Motohashi, PhD

SERIES: New Developments in Medical Research

BOOK DESCRIPTION: This book will focus on plant ingredients and plants that can be expected to maintain health until this longevity.

SOFTCOVER ISBN: 978-1-53616-282-0
RETAIL PRICE: $195

BIOCOMPOSITES IN BIO-MEDICINE

EDITORS: Mudasir Ahmad, Mohmmad Younus Wani, PhD, Preeti Singh, Saiqa Ikram, and Baoliang Zhang

SERIES: New Developments in Medical Research

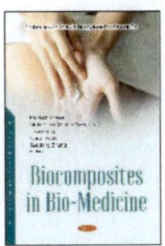

BOOK DESCRIPTION: This book covers important topics of Biopolymers nanocomposites in simple language with clear presentation. Traces of their use as biomedical and pharmaceutical application, gelatin, polysacharides based nanocomposites for applications in antibacterial/microbial/biomedical engineering, drug delivery system and tissue engineering is covered.

SOFTCOVER ISBN: 978-1-53616-247-9
RETAIL PRICE: $95

To see a complete list of Nova publications, please visit our website at www.novapublishers.com

Related Nova Publications

Oregano: Properties, Uses and Health Benefits

Editor: Gema Nieto Martínez

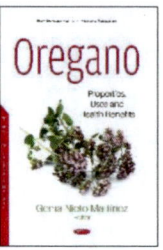

Series: New Developments in Medical Research

Book Description: This book reviews and discusses oregano containing several potent antimicrobial, antioxidant compounds that may contribute to benefit the nervous and cardiovascular systems. In addition, the opportunity of using Origanum vulgare as potential platform for producing polyphenols, biogas and energy under biorefinery approach has been discussed.

Hardcover ISBN: 978-1-53616-284-4
Retail Price: $230

Advances in Medicinal Chemistry Research

Editor: Edeildo Ferreira da Silva-Júnior

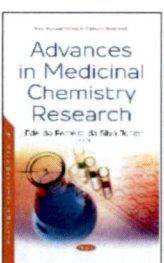

Series: New Developments in Medical Research

Book Description: *Advances in Medicinal Chemistry Research* is a book addressed to undergraduate and postgraduate students, where recent advances in the discovery and development of effective agents against the most remarkable wide-reaching diseases are presented, divided into seven chapters.

Hardcover ISBN: 978-1-53616-368-1
Retail Price: $195

To see a complete list of Nova publications, please visit our website at www.novapublishers.com